GASTRIC BYPASS COOKBOOK

FOR BEGINNERS

Delicious and Nutritious Recipes for Every Stage of Your Recovery Journey

Kingsley Klopp

SPECIAL BONUS

To show our appreciation for your purchase, we're delighted to offer you these special bonuses as a heartfelt thank you.

1. A Food Tracker Journal
2. Downloadable E-BOOK featuring full-color images of finished recipes
3. One year weight loss journal

Copyright © 2024 All rights reserved.
No part of this book may be reproduced or transmitted in any form or by any means, electronic or mechanical, including photocopying, recording, or by any information storage and retrieval system, without written permission from the author. The scanning, uploading, and distribution of this book via the internet or via any other means without the permission of the author is illegal and punishable by law. The author has made every effort to ensure the accuracy of the information contained in this book. However, the author cannot be held responsible for any errors or omissions.

Table of Contents

Introduction..7

Chapter 1
Understanding Gastric Bypass Surgery
- What is Gastric Bypass Surgery?..9
- Benefits and Risks...11
- The Recovery Process..13
- Dietary Stages Post-Surgery..15

Chapter 2
Nutrition Basics for Gastric Bypass Patients
- Macronutrients and Micronutrients..19
- Protein: The Key Nutrient...22
- Importance of Hydration..25

Clear Liquid Recipes

Homemade Chicken Broth..27
Vegetable Broth..28
Beef Broth..28
White Grape Juice..29
Mint Tea...29
Clear Iced Tea...30
Chicken Gelatin..30
Japanese Clear Soup (Osumashi)..31
Orange-Earl Grey Iced Tea...31
Blackberry Mint Iced Tea..32
Iced Peach Ginger Tea..33
Raspberry Leaf Tea...33
Licorice Tea..34

Full Liquid Recipes

Smooth Cream of Wheat..35
Blended Pumpkin Soup..36
Mashed Potato Soup...36
Pea Soup..37
Banana Smoothie...37

Avocado Smoothie..38
Pear & Ricotta Puree...38
Shrimp Scampi Puree..39
Yogurt Smoothie..39
Malted Milk Drink...40
Rice Congee..40
Egg Custard..41
Strained Cream Soups..42
Honeydew Melon Juice...42

Semisolids/Soft Foods Reipes
Mashed Sweet Potatoes..43
Refried Beans...44
Oatmeal..44
Cream of Rice...45
Banana Puree...45
Fluffy Egg Whites...46
Soft Cheesecake...46
Baba Ghanoush..47
Protein Pancakes..47
Corned Beef..48
Apple Crumbled Ramekins...48
Patty Pan Squash...49
Queso Chicken..49
Savory Quinoa Muffins...50
Greek Turkey Burgers...51
Ruby French Dressing..52

Breakfast Recipes
Greek Yogurt with Mashed Berries...53
Protein Powder Porridge..54
Silken Tofu Scramble...54
Savory Mashed Pumpkin..55
Creamed Barley..55
Vegetable Juice Smoothie..56
Kefir with Pureed Mango..56
Low-fat Quark Cheese..57
Butternut Squash and Apple Mash...57
Carrot and Zucchini Bread Pudding...58
Protein Enriched Apple Smoothie..59
Steamed Vegetable Puree...59
Sweet Potato Puree..60
Soy Yogurt Parfait..60
Acorn Squash Puree...61

Soft Papaya Mash...62
Low-fat Milk Porridge..62
Liquidized Porridge Pancakes...63

Poultry & Meat Recipes
Ground Turkey Soup..64
Soft Cooked Chicken Thighs..65
Pulled Pork...66
Beef Tenderloin Puree..67
Pork Tenderloin Mousse..68
Chicken Liver Pate..69
Protein-rich Turkey Broth...70
Meat Jello..71
Soft Poached Chicken Breast..72
Ground Beef Stew...73
Tender Beef Goulash..74
Ground Lamb Soup..75
Chicken with Mushrooms...76
Blackened Chicken Breast...77
Mexicali Meatloaf..78
Chinese Pork..79
Wiener Schnitzel...80
Soft Meatballs in Tomato Sauce...81
Tender Veal Stew..82
Silky Turkey Gravy...83
Chicken Crepe Filling..83
Mild Meat Chili...84
Pureed Liver with Onion..85
Tender Stewed Rabbit..86
Chicken and Yogurt Soup...87

Fish and Seafood Recipes
Pureed White Fish..88
Soft Salmon Mousse...89
Tender Flaked Tuna..89
Paprika Shrimp Puree..90
Silky Lobster Bisque...90
Sole in White Sauce..91
Scallop Pate..91
Mashed Anchovies...92
Tilapia Puree..92

Creamy Salmon Spread...93
Flounder and Parsley Soup..93
Shrimp and Cucumber Gel..94
Mild Mackerel Puree...95
Tuna and Sweet Potato Mash..95
Catfish Soup...96
Haddock in Mustard Sauce...97
Barramundi Broth...97
Snapper and Carrot Soup...98
Mullet in Light Broth..98
Crawfish Tail Mix..99

Soup & Stew Recipes
Chicken and Thyme Broth..100
Turkey and Sage Soup...101
Lentil and Ham Soup..101
Pea and Mint Soup...102
Silky Egg Drop Soup...103
Quinoa and Vegetable Stew..104
Venison Broth...104
Duck and Ginger Broth...105
Rabbit and Herb Soup..105
Bison and Vegetable Broth...106
Spinach and Chicken Soup..106
Pheasant Soup..107
Soft Cod Soup...107
Smooth Asparagus and Turkey Soup...108
Parsnip and Pork Soup...108
Cauliflower and Cod Stew..109
Tender Goat Meat Stew..109
Chicken Gizzard Soup..110

Desserts & Snacks
Coconut Milk Rice Pudding..111
Caramel Protein Mousse..112
Peaches and Cream Protein Smoothie..112
Soft Baked Protein Apple Slices...113
Chocolate Hazelnut Spread..114
Maple Almond Protein Custard..115
Pumpkin Spice Soft Cookies..116
Soft Carrot Cake Squares...116
Protein Flan..117
Low-fat Tiramisu...117

Creamy Banana Soft Serve..118
Cacao Nib Protein Yogurt..118
Fluffy Protein Pancakes..119

8-Week Meal Plan...120

Introduction

Welcome to a transformative journey towards a healthier, more vibrant you. If you've picked up this book, chances are you've made the life-changing decision to undergo gastric bypass surgery, or you're considering it. Either way, congratulations! You're embarking on a path that promises not just weight loss, but a complete overhaul of your well-being. But let's be honest – the road ahead isn't just paved with good intentions; it's lined with dietary changes, lifestyle adjustments, and a whole lot of learning. That's where this **Gastric Bypass Cookbook for Beginners** comes in.

I remember the first day after my own gastric bypass surgery. The excitement of a new beginning was mixed with a whirlwind of questions. What can I eat? How much can I eat? How do I make sure I'm getting the right nutrients? It was overwhelming. If you're feeling the same way, take a deep breath. This cookbook is here to guide you every step of the way, from your first sip of broth to enjoying a wholesome, balanced meal. Let's face it – food is more than just fuel for our bodies. It's a source of comfort, a way to celebrate, and a means to connect with others. The prospect of changing your eating habits can feel daunting, but it doesn't have to be a struggle. With the right tools, knowledge, and a little creativity, you'll discover that eating after gastric bypass can be both delicious and satisfying. This book isn't just a collection of recipes; it's a comprehensive guide to your new culinary life. We'll start with the basics, covering the essential information about gastric bypass surgery, what to expect in the days and weeks following the procedure, and how to navigate the different phases of your new diet. You'll learn about the nutritional needs that are unique to gastric bypass patients, and how to meet them without feeling deprived or overwhelmed. Each chapter is designed to build your confidence in the kitchen, from preparing simple, nutrient-dense meals to experimenting with more adventurous dishes. You'll find tips on meal planning, portion control, and mindful eating – all critical components of your success. And because life doesn't stop after surgery, there are also practical strategies for dining out, traveling, and managing social situations.

One of the most exciting aspects of this journey is discovering new foods and flavors that you might not have considered before. This cookbook features a diverse array of recipes, from hearty breakfasts to savory dinners and everything in between. Whether you're a novice cook or a seasoned chef, you'll find inspiration and guidance here. Remember, this isn't just about losing weight; it's about gaining a new lease on life. The changes you're making now will have far-reaching benefits, improving your overall health, energy levels, and self-esteem. You're not alone on this path – consider this cookbook your friendly companion, ready to offer support, encouragement, and delicious recipes that make your journey enjoyable.

So, are you ready to take the first step towards a healthier, happier you? Let's dive in and start cooking up a storm. Welcome to your new, flavorful, and nourishing world!

Understanding Gastric Bypass Surgery

What is Gastric Bypass Surgery?

Gastric bypass surgery is a transformative procedure, often representing a new lease on life for those battling severe obesity. It's not just a surgical intervention; it's a profound step toward reclaiming one's health, vitality, and overall well-being. For many, this surgery is a beacon of hope after years of struggling with weight-related issues, failed diets, and health complications. At its core, gastric bypass surgery involves making changes to your digestive system to help you lose weight. This procedure is typically reserved for individuals who have not been able to achieve significant weight loss through diet and exercise and are dealing with serious health problems due to obesity, such as type 2 diabetes, high blood pressure, or heart disease. The process begins with the surgeon creating a small stomach pouch, about the size of a walnut, out of the existing stomach. This significantly reduces the amount of food one can eat at any given time, which helps in limiting calorie intake. The surgeon then connects this newly created pouch directly to a section of the small intestine, bypassing a large part of the stomach and the initial segment of the small intestine. This bypass reduces the absorption of calories and nutrients, contributing to weight loss.

Understanding the mechanics of gastric bypass surgery is crucial, but it's equally important to grasp the emotional journey involved. The decision to undergo this surgery is often the result of years of contemplation, soul-searching, and sometimes, desperation. Many individuals have tried countless diets, experienced the pain of failure, and dealt with the societal stigma attached to obesity. Gastric bypass surgery offers a chance for a fresh start, but it's not a decision taken lightly. It's a commitment to a new way of living, one that requires significant lifestyle changes, dedication, and resilience. Post-surgery, patients often experience rapid weight loss, which can be both exhilarating and overwhelming. Shedding pounds can lead to improved mobility, increased energy levels, and a dramatic reduction in obesity-related health issues. Imagine the joy of walking without pain, the thrill of being able to engage in activities that were once out of reach, and the profound relief of seeing improvements in health metrics. It's like being handed the keys to a future that once seemed unattainable.

However, this journey is not without its challenges. The physical recovery from surgery is just the beginning. Patients must adapt to new eating habits, often dealing with discomfort as their body adjusts. The emotional aspect of adjusting to a new self-image can be equally demanding. Support from healthcare professionals, family, and support groups is vital during this period. The emotional support helps patients navigate the highs and lows, celebrating victories and managing setbacks with a sense of community and understanding. Moreover, gastric bypass surgery necessitates lifelong changes in how one approaches food and nutrition. It's a transition from viewing food as a source of comfort to seeing it as fuel for the body. This shift in perspective can be liberating but also requires a continuous effort to maintain. Regular follow-ups with healthcare providers, adhering to a nutritious diet, taking prescribed supplements, and staying active are all part of the ongoing commitment to health.

The transformative power of gastric bypass surgery extends beyond physical health. It can lead to improved mental health, higher self-esteem, and a more positive outlook on life. The journey toward health is filled with milestones, each step forward building confidence and reinforcing the belief that a healthier, happier life is within reach.

Benefits and Risks of Gastric Bypass Surgery

Benefits
One of the most compelling benefits of gastric bypass surgery is substantial weight loss. For many individuals, this procedure represents a breakthrough after years of unsuccessful dieting and exercise attempts. By reducing the stomach's size and altering the digestive process, patients often experience rapid and sustained weight loss. This reduction in body weight can lead to dramatic improvements in overall health.

Improved Health Outcomes: One of the most significant advantages of gastric bypass surgery is its impact on obesity-related health conditions. Patients frequently see a reversal or significant improvement in conditions such as type 2 diabetes, hypertension, sleep apnea, and high cholesterol. For many, this means reducing or even eliminating the need for medication, leading to a better quality of life and increased longevity.

Enhanced Mobility and Activity Levels: As the weight comes off, patients often find that they can move more freely and engage in physical activities that were previously too difficult or painful. This increase in activity further contributes to weight loss and helps build muscle strength and cardiovascular health.

Psychological Benefits: Beyond the physical changes, gastric bypass surgery can profoundly affect mental health. Many patients report increased self-esteem and confidence as they reach their weight loss goals. The psychological relief from achieving a healthier body weight can alleviate symptoms of depression and anxiety, providing a more positive outlook on life.

Risks
Despite these considerable benefits, gastric bypass surgery is not without its risks. It is a major surgical procedure that requires a commitment to lifelong changes in diet and lifestyle.

Surgical Complications: As with any major surgery, there are risks associated with the procedure itself. These include infections, blood clots, and adverse reactions to anesthesia. More specific to gastric bypass, there can be complications such as leaks in the gastrointestinal tract, which require immediate medical attention.

Nutritional Deficiencies: Since the surgery alters the digestive process, it can lead to malabsorption of essential nutrients. Patients must adhere to a strict regimen of vitamins and supplements to prevent deficiencies in calcium, iron, vitamin B12, and other critical nutrients. Failure to do so can result in long-term health issues like osteoporosis, anemia, and neurological problems.

Dumping Syndrome: A common side effect of gastric bypass surgery is dumping syndrome, where food moves too quickly from the stomach to the small intestine. This can cause symptoms such as nausea, vomiting, diarrhea, and dizziness. Managing dumping syndrome requires careful attention to diet, avoiding high-sugar and high-fat foods.

Weight Regain: While gastric bypass surgery offers a tool for significant weight loss, it is not a guarantee. Without commitment to a healthy lifestyle, including regular exercise and proper nutrition, there is a risk of weight regain. The surgery requires a permanent change in eating habits and ongoing behavioral therapy to maintain the benefits.

Emotional and Psychological Challenges: Adjusting to the new body and lifestyle can be challenging. Some patients may struggle with changes in self-image and relationships. Access to counseling and support groups can help navigate these emotional transitions.

In summary, gastric bypass surgery offers profound benefits, particularly for individuals struggling with severe obesity and related health conditions. However, it also carries risks that require careful consideration and a commitment to long-term lifestyle changes. By weighing these benefits and risks, patients can make informed decisions about whether gastric bypass surgery is the right path for their health journey.

The Recovery Process

The recovery process after gastric bypass surgery is a journey of transformation, resilience, and hope. It marks the beginning of a new chapter, filled with challenges and triumphs as individuals reclaim their health and well-being. This period is crucial, not only for physical healing but also for adapting to a new lifestyle that ensures long-term success.

Immediate Post-Surgery Phase

Immediately after surgery, patients awaken in the recovery room, surrounded by the steady beeping of monitors and the reassuring presence of medical staff. There's a mix of relief and anticipation as the first step of this life-changing journey is complete. Pain and discomfort are common initially, but modern pain management techniques and medications help alleviate these sensations. Nurses frequently check on the patient's vitals, ensuring that everything is progressing smoothly.

During the first few days, the focus is on healing and avoiding complications. Patients are encouraged to take short, gentle walks around the hospital to stimulate blood flow and reduce the risk of blood clots. Though these first steps may seem daunting, they are vital for a smooth recovery. The body's resilience is remarkable, and each movement, however small, contributes to the healing process.

Dietary Adjustments

The journey of adapting to new dietary habits begins in the hospital. Initially, patients are restricted to clear liquids to give their stomach time to heal. This phase can be emotionally challenging, as the familiar comforts of solid food are temporarily out of reach. However, this stage is essential for ensuring that the stomach and intestines recover properly.

As days turn into weeks, patients gradually transition from clear liquids to full liquids, then to pureed foods, and eventually to soft foods. This progression is carefully monitored by healthcare providers to ensure that the new stomach structure can handle different types of nourishment. It's a period of rediscovery, where patients learn to savor small, nutrient-dense meals and listen to their body's cues of fullness and satisfaction.

Physical and Emotional Adaptation

Recovery from gastric bypass surgery is as much an emotional journey as it is a physical one. The rapid weight loss that follows the surgery can bring about a whirlwind of emotions—joy, relief, and even anxiety. The reflection in the mirror starts to change, and with it, self-perception. Support from family, friends, and support groups becomes invaluable during this time. Sharing experiences with others who have undergone the same surgery can provide comfort, encouragement, and practical advice.

Physically, the body adjusts to the new digestive system. Patients must learn to eat slowly, chew thoroughly, and avoid foods that may cause discomfort or "dumping syndrome," where food moves too quickly through the stomach and intestines, leading to nausea and dizziness. Regular follow-ups with healthcare providers help monitor progress and address any complications that may arise.

Long-Term Recovery and Lifestyle Changes

As recovery progresses, the focus shifts to long-term health and lifestyle changes. Regular physical activity becomes a cornerstone of the new routine. Exercise not only aids in weight loss but also enhances mood, energy levels, and overall well-being. Patients often find joy in activities that were previously too strenuous, such as walking, swimming, or even participating in fitness classes.

Nutrition remains a lifelong priority. Patients work with dietitians to develop meal plans that ensure adequate protein intake and prevent nutritional deficiencies. This period involves experimenting with different foods, discovering new recipes, and learning to enjoy a balanced diet that supports ongoing health goals.

Embracing a New Life

The recovery process after gastric bypass surgery is transformative. It's a period of profound change, where individuals redefine their relationship with food, their body, and their overall health. The journey is marked by milestones—losing the first significant amount of weight, fitting into smaller clothes, receiving positive feedback from loved ones, and achieving health improvements that once seemed impossible.

Throughout this journey, patience and perseverance are key. There will be moments of struggle and moments of triumph, but each step forward brings a renewed sense of hope and possibility. Gastric bypass surgery is not just about losing weight; it's about gaining a new lease on life. It's about finding the strength to overcome challenges, celebrating progress, and embracing a healthier, happier future.

Dietary Stages Post-Surgery

The journey to health and wellness after gastric bypass surgery is structured around several critical dietary stages. Each stage plays a vital role in ensuring proper healing, adapting to new eating habits, and promoting sustained weight loss. Adhering to these stages helps prevent complications, ensures adequate nutrition, and supports long-term success.

Stage 1: Clear Liquids
Duration: 1-2 days
Purpose: The clear liquids stage immediately follows the surgery and serves to allow the stomach and intestines to heal without the stress of digestion. This stage helps prevent dehydration and prepares the body for subsequent dietary stages.
What to Consume:
- Water
- Broth (chicken, beef, or vegetable)
- Sugar-free gelatin
- Decaffeinated tea
- Sugar-free popsicles
- Electrolyte drinks (low-calorie)

Guidelines:
- Sip slowly and continuously throughout the day.
- Aim for at least 64 ounces of fluids per day.
- Avoid caffeine, sugar, and carbonation.

Stage 2: Full Liquids
Duration: 1-2 weeks
Purpose: This stage introduces more nutrition while still minimizing strain on the digestive system. It includes liquids that are slightly more substantial than clear liquids.
What to Consume:
- Protein shakes (low-sugar)
- Strained cream soups (blended without chunks)
- Low-fat yogurt (without fruit chunks)
- Milk (skim or 1%)
- Sugar-free pudding
- Smooth, low-fat cottage cheese

Guidelines:
- Continue to stay hydrated with at least 64 ounces of fluids daily.
- Introduce protein-rich liquids to meet protein goals (usually 60-80 grams per day).
- Avoid sugary and fatty liquids.

Stage 3: Pureed Foods
Duration: 2-4 weeks
Purpose: The pureed foods stage is designed to reintroduce more solid foods in a form that is easy to digest and gentle on the healing stomach. It provides essential nutrients and helps patients adjust to consuming more varied foods.
What to Consume:
- Pureed lean meats (chicken, turkey, fish)
- Pureed vegetables (carrots, peas, green beans)
- Mashed potatoes
- Unsweetened applesauce
- Pureed fruits (bananas, pears)
- Scrambled eggs (blended to a smooth consistency)

Guidelines:
- Puree foods to a smooth, pudding-like consistency.
- Eat small, frequent meals (5-6 times per day).
- Chew food thoroughly even though it's pureed to aid digestion.
- Focus on protein intake and avoid fibrous, tough, or crunchy foods.

Stage 4: Soft Foods
Duration: 4-6 weeks
Purpose: This stage further transitions patients to more regular textures while ensuring that the foods are soft enough not to disrupt healing.
What to Consume:
- Ground or finely chopped meats (chicken, turkey, fish)
- Soft fruits (banana, canned fruits in natural juice)
- Soft cooked vegetables (zucchini, squash, green beans)
- Low-fat cheese
- Soft-cooked eggs
- Tofu

Guidelines:
- Continue eating small, frequent meals.
- Chew food thoroughly until it reaches a paste-like consistency.
- Introduce new foods one at a time to monitor tolerance.
- Avoid raw vegetables, crunchy foods, and tough meats.

Stage 5: Solid Foods
Duration: 6+ weeks post-surgery
Purpose: The solid foods stage marks the return to a more typical diet, though portion sizes are permanently smaller, and food choices remain focused on supporting weight loss and overall health.
What to Consume:
- Lean proteins (chicken, turkey, fish, lean beef)
- Whole grains (quinoa, brown rice, whole grain bread)
- Fresh fruits (in moderation)
- Vegetables (raw and cooked)
- Low-fat dairy products
- Healthy fats (avocado, olive oil, nuts in small quantities)

Guidelines:
- Maintain a focus on protein intake (60-80 grams per day).
- Eat balanced meals that include a variety of nutrients.
- Continue to avoid high-sugar, high-fat, and high-carb foods.
- Keep portions small and monitor for any discomfort or intolerance.
- Stay hydrated, drinking fluids between meals but not with meals to avoid overfilling the stomach.

Long-Term Maintenance
Purpose: Long-term maintenance involves sustaining the dietary habits developed during the post-surgery stages to ensure continued weight loss and health benefits.
What to Focus On:
- Balanced meals with lean protein, vegetables, and whole grains.
- Regular physical activity to support weight loss and overall health.
- Continued monitoring of portion sizes.
- Avoidance of "slider foods" (high-calorie, easily digestible foods that can sabotage weight loss).
- Routine follow-ups with healthcare providers and dietitians.

Guidelines:
- Develop a consistent meal routine.
- Prioritize nutrient-dense foods to meet dietary needs without excess calories.
- Stay mindful of emotional eating and seek support if needed.
- Continue taking recommended vitamins and supplements to prevent deficiencies.

The dietary stages post-gastric bypass surgery are designed to promote healing, ensure proper nutrition, and establish healthy eating habits that will support long-term weight management and overall well-being. This journey requires commitment, patience, and a willingness to embrace new ways of eating. Each stage is a step towards a healthier, more fulfilling life, with the ultimate goal of achieving sustained weight loss and improved quality of life. Through careful adherence to these stages, individuals can maximize the benefits of their surgery and enjoy the profound health transformations that follow.

Macronutrients and Micronutrients

Macronutrients
Macronutrients are the nutrients required in large amounts in the diet. They include proteins, carbohydrates, and fats. Each plays a critical role in bodily functions and overall well-being.

1. Protein
Importance:
- Protein is the cornerstone of post-gastric bypass nutrition. It is essential for tissue repair, muscle maintenance, and overall healing.
- Adequate protein intake helps prevent muscle loss, a common concern after significant weight loss.

Sources:
- Lean meats (chicken, turkey, fish)
- Low-fat dairy products (yogurt, cottage cheese, milk)
- Eggs
- Legumes and beans
- Protein supplements (whey, soy, or pea protein)

Guidelines:
- Aim for 60-80 grams of protein per day.
- Prioritize protein in every meal and snack.
- Use protein shakes or powders to meet daily protein requirements, especially in the initial stages post-surgery when solid food intake is limited.

2. Carbohydrates
Importance:
- Carbohydrates are the body's primary energy source. They fuel the brain, muscles, and other vital organs.
- However, the type and amount of carbohydrates consumed should be carefully managed post-surgery to avoid weight regain and dumping syndrome.

Sources:
- Whole grains (quinoa, brown rice, whole wheat bread)
- Vegetables (broccoli, spinach, carrots)
- Fruits (berries, apples, pears)

Guidelines:
- Focus on complex carbohydrates that provide fiber and essential nutrients.
- Limit intake of simple sugars and refined carbs, which can cause blood sugar spikes and contribute to dumping syndrome.
- Include a small portion of healthy carbohydrates in each meal to balance energy levels and promote satiety.

3. Fats
Importance:
- Fats are essential for hormone production, nutrient absorption, and cell health.
- Healthy fats provide long-lasting energy and help keep skin, hair, and nails healthy.

Sources:
- Avocado
- Nuts and seeds (in moderation)
- Olive oil
- Fatty fish (salmon, mackerel)

Guidelines:
- Choose unsaturated fats over saturated and trans fats.
- Limit fat intake to 20-35% of daily calories.
- Avoid fried foods and high-fat processed snacks, which can be difficult to digest and lead to weight regain.

Micronutrients

Micronutrients are vitamins and minerals required in smaller amounts but are equally vital for health. Gastric bypass surgery can impact the absorption of these nutrients, making supplementation and careful dietary planning essential.

1. Vitamins

Vitamin B12:
- Essential for red blood cell formation, neurological function, and DNA synthesis.
- Absorption is significantly impacted by gastric bypass surgery.

Sources:
- Animal products (meat, fish, dairy)
- Fortified foods
- Supplements (often necessary)

Vitamin D:
- Crucial for bone health and immune function.
- Limited sun exposure and dietary intake can necessitate supplementation.

Sources:
- Fatty fish
- Fortified dairy products
- Supplements

Vitamin A:
- Important for vision, immune function, and skin health.

Sources:
- Liver
- Fish oils
- Carrots and leafy green vegetables

2. Minerals

Calcium:
- Vital for bone health and muscle function.
- Absorption can be reduced post-surgery, increasing the risk of osteoporosis.

Sources:
- Dairy products
- Leafy green vegetables
- Fortified foods
- Supplements

Iron:
- Necessary for oxygen transport in the blood.
- Risk of deficiency increases post-surgery due to reduced stomach acid and bypassed intestines.

Sources:
- Red meat
- Beans and lentils
- Fortified cereals
- Supplements

Zinc:
- Important for immune function, wound healing, and protein synthesis.

Sources:
- Meat and shellfish
- Nuts and seeds
- Dairy products

Magnesium:
- Involved in over 300 biochemical reactions in the body, including energy production and bone health.

Sources:
- Nuts and seeds
- Leafy green vegetables
- Whole grains

Nutritional Supplementation

Due to the malabsorptive nature of gastric bypass surgery, patients are often advised to take specific supplements to prevent deficiencies. A typical regimen includes:

- **Multivitamin:** A high-potency multivitamin to cover basic needs.
- **Calcium Citrate:** Preferred over calcium carbonate for better absorption post-surgery, usually taken in divided doses.
- **Vitamin B12:** Often required as a sublingual tablet, nasal spray, or injection.
- **Iron and Vitamin C:** Iron supplementation is often paired with vitamin C to enhance absorption.
- **Vitamin D:** Taken in conjunction with calcium to support bone health.

Protein: The Key Nutrient

Protein is often hailed as the cornerstone of nutrition, especially for those who have undergone gastric bypass surgery. This essential macronutrient plays a crucial role in recovery, weight management, and overall health. Understanding the importance of protein, its sources, and how to incorporate it effectively into the diet is vital for anyone navigating life after gastric bypass surgery.

The Importance of Protein Post-Gastric Bypass

1. Healing and Tissue Repair
- After gastric bypass surgery, your body is like a wounded warrior in need of repair. Protein is the building block that helps mend the tissues and heal the surgical wounds. It's the fuel that powers your recovery, allowing you to rebuild and regain strength.

2. Maintaining Muscle Mass
- Rapid weight loss can be a double-edged sword. While shedding excess pounds is a victory, losing muscle mass is a potential pitfall. Protein is your ally in preserving muscle mass, which is crucial for maintaining strength, metabolism, and overall physical function. Muscle mass not only supports your metabolic rate but also empowers you to stay active and vibrant.

3. Supporting Immune Function
- Your immune system is your body's defense mechanism, and protein is vital for its proper functioning. Post-surgery, your body is vulnerable, and protein helps produce antibodies and immune cells that protect you from infections and illnesses. It's like having an army ready to defend your newfound health.

4. Satiety and Weight Management
- One of protein's superpowers is its ability to keep you feeling full and satisfied. This is a game-changer for managing hunger and preventing overeating. Protein helps you adhere to the smaller portion sizes required after surgery, making it easier to stay on track with your weight management goals.

5. Preventing Hair Loss
- Hair loss can be a distressing side effect of rapid weight loss and nutritional deficiencies. Protein provides the nutrients necessary for healthy hair, helping to mitigate this issue and maintain your confidence during your transformation.

Recommended Protein Intake

Post-gastric bypass patients are generally advised to consume between 60-80 grams of protein per day. This requirement can vary based on individual factors such as weight, activity level, and overall health. Meeting this protein goal is critical for the reasons mentioned above and can be challenging given the reduced stomach size and altered digestion.

Sources of Protein

1. Lean Meats
- Chicken, turkey, and fish are excellent sources of lean protein. These should be prepared in ways that avoid added fats, such as grilling, baking, or steaming, ensuring they are both nutritious and easy on your new stomach.

2. Dairy Products
- Low-fat or non-fat dairy products like Greek yogurt, cottage cheese, and milk are rich in protein. They are usually well-tolerated and easy to digest, providing a comforting and nutritious option.

3. Eggs
- Eggs are a versatile and highly nutritious source of protein. Whether scrambled, boiled, or poached, they offer a gentle and effective way to meet your protein needs.

4. Legumes and Beans
- Beans, lentils, and chickpeas provide not only protein but also fiber, which is beneficial for digestive health. These can be added to soups, salads, or pureed for easier digestion, offering variety and nutritional benefits.

5. Protein Supplements
- Protein shakes and powders (whey, soy, or pea protein) are often necessary to meet daily protein goals, especially in the early stages post-surgery when solid food intake is limited. These supplements should be low in sugar and fat to avoid unnecessary calories, providing a convenient and effective solution.

6. Seafood
- Fish and shellfish, such as salmon, tuna, and shrimp, are not only high in protein but also contain healthy fats like omega-3 fatty acids, which are beneficial for heart health. These options add flavor and nutritional value to your diet.

Incorporating Protein into the Diet

1. Meal Planning
- Plan your meals around protein sources. Start with the protein portion and build the meal with vegetables and whole grains to ensure a balanced and nutrient-dense diet. This approach helps prioritize protein intake and maintain nutritional balance.

2. Small, Frequent Meals
- Post-surgery, eating small, frequent meals is crucial. Incorporating protein into each meal and snack helps meet your daily protein requirement without overloading your digestive system, ensuring a steady supply of this essential nutrient.

3. Chewing Thoroughly
- Chew protein-rich foods thoroughly to aid digestion and prevent discomfort. This is especially important for meats and fibrous proteins, ensuring they are broken down adequately for your altered digestive system.

4. Protein First
- Eat protein first at each meal to ensure you meet your protein needs before filling up on other foods. This strategy helps prioritize protein intake and manage satiety, keeping you on track with your nutritional goals.

5. Tracking Intake
- Keeping a food diary or using a nutrition app to track protein intake can be helpful. This ensures that you are meeting your protein goals consistently, providing a sense of accomplishment and reassurance.

Potential Challenges and Solutions

1. Taste Fatigue
- Eating the same protein sources repeatedly can lead to taste fatigue. Varied preparation methods and incorporating different spices and herbs can keep meals interesting and palatable, making it easier to stick to your protein goals.

2. Digestive Issues
- Some patients may experience digestive issues with certain protein sources. Experimenting with different types of proteins and preparation methods can help identify the most tolerable options, ensuring a comfortable and enjoyable diet.

3. Accessibility and Convenience
- Preparing high-protein meals can sometimes be time-consuming. Pre-cooking and portioning protein-rich foods, or using ready-to-eat options like protein shakes, can make it easier to stick to your dietary plan, providing convenience and consistency.

The Importance of Hydration

The Role of Hydration in Post-Surgery Recovery
1. Healing and Tissue Repair
- Water is the essence of life, fueling every cell, every tissue, and every process within our bodies. After gastric bypass surgery, your body is working overtime to heal and repair. Adequate hydration is essential for transporting nutrients and oxygen to cells, accelerating the healing process and helping you get back on your feet.

2. Digestive Health
- Imagine your digestive system as a complex, finely-tuned machine. Water is the lubricant that keeps this machine running smoothly. Proper hydration aids digestion and nutrient absorption, helping to prevent the discomfort of constipation and dehydration, common challenges after surgery.

3. Kidney Function
- Your kidneys are your body's natural filtration system, and they rely on water to function effectively. Staying hydrated helps flush out toxins and prevent kidney stones, a risk that can be heightened after gastric bypass surgery due to changes in calcium and oxalate metabolism.

Challenges of Staying Hydrated Post-Surgery
1. Reduced Stomach Capacity
- With a smaller stomach, the simple act of drinking water becomes a balancing act. You can no longer gulp down large amounts; instead, you must learn to sip slowly and consistently throughout the day, a small but significant change in your daily routine.

2. Avoiding Fluid During Meals
- To maximize nutrient absorption and avoid overfilling your stomach, you need to separate drinking from eating. This means no fluids 30 minutes before and after meals, making it even more challenging to stay hydrated but crucial for your health.

3. Sensitivity to Temperature and Texture
- Post-surgery, you might find that certain temperatures or textures of fluids are more tolerable than others. This newfound sensitivity can make drinking enough water feel like a daunting task, but finding what works best for you can make all the difference.

Benefits of Proper Hydration
1. Weight Loss Support
- Drinking water can actually aid in your weight loss journey. Sometimes, your body confuses thirst with hunger, leading you to eat when you simply need to hydrate. By staying hydrated, you can better manage your appetite and support your weight loss goals.

2. Skin Health
- Hydration is key to maintaining healthy, elastic skin. As your body changes rapidly with weight loss, staying hydrated helps your skin adapt, reducing the appearance of sagging and keeping it vibrant.

3. Energy Levels
- Dehydration can sap your energy and leave you feeling fatigued. By keeping your body well-hydrated, you can maintain your energy levels, supporting an active lifestyle that is crucial for continued weight loss and health.

Practical Tips for Maintaining Hydration

1. Sip Throughout the Day
- Carry a water bottle with you and make sipping a habit. Small, frequent sips are easier for your new stomach to handle and will help keep you hydrated throughout the day.

2. Set Hydration Goals
- Aim for at least 64 ounces of fluids daily. Setting specific hydration goals and tracking your intake can make meeting your needs a more manageable and satisfying accomplishment.

3. Use Hydration Aids
- Sometimes plain water can feel monotonous. Sugar-free flavored water, herbal teas, and electrolyte drinks can add variety and make hydration more enjoyable. Just remember to avoid caffeinated and carbonated beverages.

4. Incorporate Hydrating Foods
- High-water-content foods like cucumbers, watermelon, and oranges can contribute to your hydration. Including these in your diet is a delicious way to supplement your fluid intake.

5. Listen to Your Body
- Pay close attention to signs of dehydration, such as dark urine, dry mouth, dizziness, and fatigue. These signals are your body's way of asking for more water, so respond with care and urgency.

6. Monitor Fluid Tolerance
- Experiment with different fluids and temperatures to find what works best for you. Whether it's warm herbal tea or chilled water, discovering your preferences can make hydration a more pleasant experience.

Addressing Hydration Barriers

1. Dealing with Nausea
- Nausea can make drinking water feel like a chore. Sipping on ginger tea or water with a splash of lemon can help ease nausea and make it easier to stay hydrated.

2. Managing Taste Changes
- Post-surgery taste changes are common. If plain water doesn't appeal to you, try infusing it with fruits like berries or citrus to enhance flavor without adding sugar or calories.

Clear Liquid Recipes

1. Homemade Chicken Broth
Ingredients:
- 1 whole chicken (about 3-4 pounds)
- 2 large carrots, peeled and cut into chunks
- 2 celery stalks, cut into chunks
- 1 large onion, peeled and quartered
- 4 garlic cloves, peeled
- 1 bay leaf
- 10 cups water
- Salt to taste
- Fresh parsley for garnish (optional)

Instructions:
1. Place the chicken in a large pot.
2. Add the carrots, celery, onion, garlic, and bay leaf.
3. Pour in the water and bring to a boil over high heat.
4. Reduce the heat to low and simmer for 3 hours, skimming off any foam that rises to the top.
5. Remove the chicken and vegetables from the broth. Discard the vegetables.
6. Strain the broth through a fine-mesh sieve into another pot or large bowl.
7. Season with salt to taste.
8. Cool the broth in the refrigerator, then skim off any fat that solidifies on the surface.

Nutrition Info (per serving):
- Calories: 80
- Protein: 10g
- Fat: 3g
- Carbohydrates: 1g
- Fiber: 0g
- Sodium: 250mg

Servings: 10 **Cooking Time:** 3 hours 15 minutes

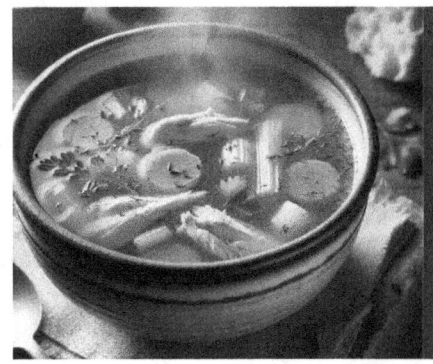

2. Vegetable Broth

Ingredients:
- 2 large carrots, peeled and chopped
- 2 celery stalks, chopped
- 1 large onion, chopped
- 2 garlic cloves, peeled
- 1 bay leaf
- 1 bunch parsley
- 10 cups water
- Salt to taste

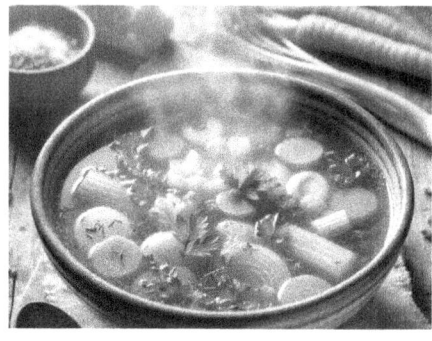

Instructions:
1. Combine all ingredients in a large pot.
2. Bring to a boil over high heat.
3. Reduce the heat to low and simmer for 1.5 hours.
4. Strain the broth through a fine-mesh sieve.
5. Season with salt to taste.

Nutrition Info (per serving):
- Calories: 20 Protein: 0g Fat: 0g Carbohydrates: 5g Fiber: 1g Sodium: 200mg

Servings: 10 **Cooking Time:** 1.5 hours

3. Beef Broth

Ingredients:
- 2 pounds beef bones
- 2 large carrots, peeled and chopped
- 2 celery stalks, chopped
- 1 large onion, chopped
- 2 garlic cloves, peeled
- 1 bay leaf
- 10 cups water
- Salt to taste

Instructions:
1. Preheat oven to 400°F (200°C).
2. Place the beef bones in a roasting pan and roast for 30 minutes.
3. Transfer the bones to a large pot.
4. Add the carrots, celery, onion, garlic, and bay leaf.
5. Pour in the water and bring to a boil over high heat.
6. Reduce the heat to low and simmer for 4 hours, skimming off any foam.
7. Strain the broth through a fine-mesh sieve.
8. Season with salt to taste.

Nutrition Info (per serving):
- Calories: 50 Protein: 5g Fat: 2g Carbohydrates: 1g Fiber: 0g Sodium: 300mg

Servings: 10 **Cooking Time:** 4 hours 30 minutes

4. White Grape Juice
Ingredients:
- 3 pounds seedless white grapes
- 1 cup water
- Sugar (optional, to taste)

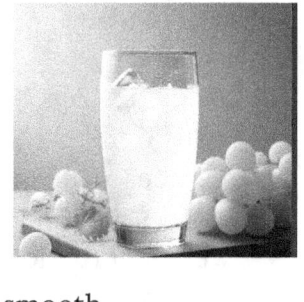

Instructions:
1. Wash the grapes thoroughly.
2. Place the grapes and water in a blender and blend until smooth.
3. Strain the mixture through a fine-mesh sieve or cheesecloth.
4. Add sugar to taste if desired.
5. Chill in the refrigerator before serving.

Nutrition Info (per serving):
- Calories: 150 Protein: 0g Fat: 0g Carbohydrates: 37g Fiber: 1g Sodium: 5mg

Servings: 6 **Cooking Time:** 15 minutes

5. Mint Tea
Ingredients:
- 1 bunch fresh mint leaves
- 4 cups water
- Honey or sweetener (optional)

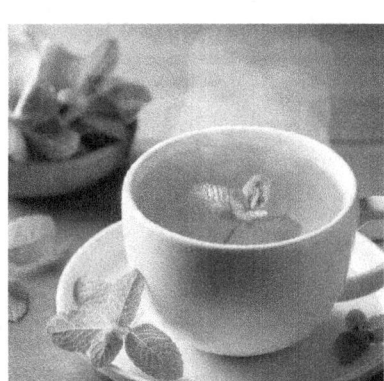

Instructions:
1. Wash the mint leaves thoroughly.
2. Boil the water in a pot.
3. Add the mint leaves to the boiling water.
4. Remove from heat and let steep for 5-10 minutes.
5. Strain the tea into a cup.
6. Add honey or sweetener if desired.

Nutrition Info (per serving):
- Calories: 0 (without honey or sweetener)
- Protein: 0g
- Fat: 0g
- Carbohydrates: 0g
- Fiber: 0g
- Sodium: 0mg

Servings: 4 **Cooking Time:** 10 minutes

6. Clear Iced Tea

Ingredients:
- 4 black tea bags
- 4 cups water
- Ice cubes
- Lemon slices (optional)
- Sweetener (optional)

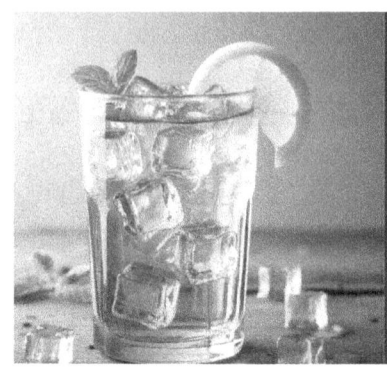

Instructions:
1. Boil the water in a pot.
2. Add the tea bags and let steep for 5 minutes.
3. Remove the tea bags and let the tea cool to room temperature.
4. Pour the tea into a pitcher and refrigerate until cold.
5. Serve over ice cubes with lemon slices and sweetener if desired.

Nutrition Info (per serving):
- Calories: 0 (without sweetener) Protein: 0g Fat: 0g Carbohydrates: 0g
- Fiber: 0g
- Sodium: 0mg

Servings: 4 **Cooking Time:** 10 minutes

7. Chicken Gelatin

Ingredients:
- 4 cups homemade chicken broth
- 2 tablespoons unflavored gelatin

Instructions:
1. Pour 1 cup of chicken broth into a small bowl.
2. Sprinkle the gelatin over the broth and let sit for 5 minutes.
3. Heat the remaining 3 cups of broth in a pot until hot but not boiling.
4. Add the gelatin mixture to the hot broth and stir until completely dissolved.
5. Pour the mixture into a dish and refrigerate until set, about 4 hours.

Nutrition Info (per serving):
- Calories: 20
- Protein: 5g
- Fat: 0g
- Carbohydrates: 0g
- Fiber: 0g
- Sodium: 300mg

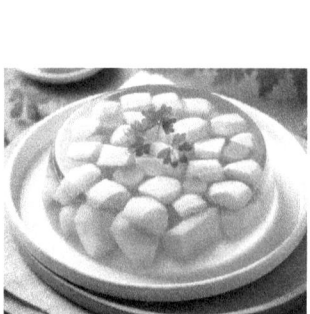

Servings: 8 **Cooking Time:** 4 hours 15 minutes

8. Japanese Clear Soup (Osumashi)

Ingredients:
- 4 cups dashi broth
- 1 tablespoon soy sauce
- 1 tablespoon mirin
- 1/2 teaspoon salt
- 1 block soft tofu, cut into small cubes
- 2 green onions, sliced thinly
- 4 shiitake mushrooms, sliced thinly
- Fresh parsley or mitsuba for garnish (optional)

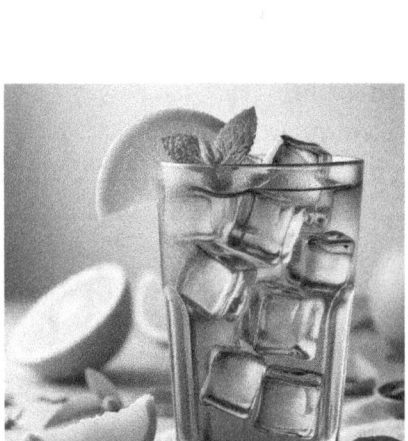

Instructions:
1. In a pot, bring the dashi broth to a boil.
2. Add the soy sauce, mirin, and salt. Stir to combine.
3. Add the tofu cubes and shiitake mushrooms. Simmer for 5 minutes.
4. Ladle the soup into bowls.
5. Garnish with sliced green onions and parsley or mitsuba if desired.

Nutrition Info (per serving):
- Calories: 40 Protein: 4g Fat: 1g Carbohydrates: 4g Fiber: 1g
- Sodium: 400mg

Servings: 4 **Cooking Time:** 15 minutes

9. Orange-Earl Grey Iced Tea

Ingredients:
- 4 Earl Grey tea bags
- 4 cups water
- 1 cup fresh orange juice
- Ice cubes
- Orange slices for garnish (optional)
- Sweetener (optional)

Instructions:
1. Boil the water in a pot.
2. Add the Earl Grey tea bags and let steep for 5 minutes.
3. Remove the tea bags and let the tea cool to room temperature.
4. Stir in the fresh orange juice.
5. Pour the tea into a pitcher and refrigerate until cold.
6. Serve over ice cubes with orange slices and sweetener if desired.

Nutrition Info (per serving):
- Calories: 25 (without sweetener) Protein: 0g Fat: 0g Carbohydrates: 6g
- Fiber: 0g
- Sodium: 0mg

Servings: 4 **Cooking Time:** 10 minutes

10. Blackberry Mint Iced Tea

Ingredients:
- 4 black tea bags
- 4 cups water
- 1 cup fresh blackberries
- 1/4 cup fresh mint leaves
- Ice cubes
- Mint sprigs and blackberries for garnish (optional)
- Sweetener (optional)

Instructions:
1. Boil the water in a pot.
2. Add the black tea bags and let steep for 5 minutes.
3. Remove the tea bags and let the tea cool to room temperature.
4. In a pitcher, muddle the fresh blackberries and mint leaves.
5. Pour the cooled tea into the pitcher and stir well.
6. Refrigerate until cold.
7. Serve over ice cubes with mint sprigs and blackberries for garnish if desired.

Nutrition Info (per serving):
- Calories: 15 (without sweetener)
- Protein: 0g
- Fat: 0g
- Carbohydrates: 4g
- Fiber: 1g
- Sodium: 0mg

Servings: 4 **Cooking Time:** 15 minutes

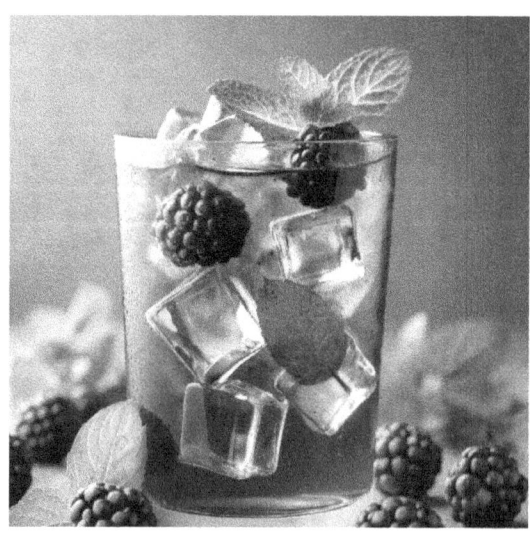

11. Iced Peach Ginger Tea

Ingredients:
- 4 green tea bags
- 4 cups water
- 2 ripe peaches, sliced
- 1-inch piece of fresh ginger, peeled and sliced
- Ice cubes
- Peach slices for garnish (optional)
- Sweetener (optional)

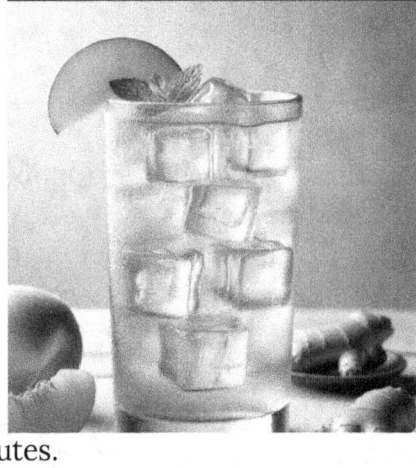

Instructions:
1. Boil the water in a pot.
2. Add the green tea bags and let steep for 5 minutes.
3. Remove the tea bags and let the tea cool to room temperature.
4. In a pitcher, add the peach slices and ginger slices.
5. Pour the cooled tea into the pitcher and stir well.
6. Refrigerate until cold.
7. Serve over ice cubes with peach slices for garnish if desired.

Nutrition Info (per serving):
Calories: 20 (without sweetener) Protein: 0g Fat: 0g Carbohydrates: 5g Fiber: 1g
- Sodium: 0mg

Servings: 4 **Cooking Time:** 15 minutes

12. Raspberry Leaf Tea

Ingredients:
- 2 tablespoons dried raspberry leaves
- 4 cups water
- Honey or sweetener (optional)

Instructions:
1. Boil the water in a pot.
2. Add the dried raspberry leaves to the boiling water.
3. Remove from heat and let steep for 10 minutes.
4. Strain the tea into a cup.
5. Add honey or sweetener if desired.

Nutrition Info (per serving):
- Calories: 0 (without honey or sweetener)
- Protein: 0g
- Fat: 0g
- Carbohydrates: 0g
- Fiber: 0g
- Sodium: 0mg

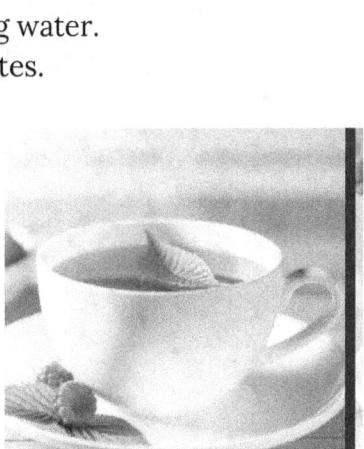

Servings: 4 **Cooking Time:** 10 minutes

13. Licorice Tea

Ingredients:
- 2 tablespoons dried licorice root
- 4 cups water
- Honey or sweetener (optional)

Instructions:
1. Boil the water in a pot.
2. Add the dried licorice root to the boiling water.
3. Remove from heat and let steep for 10 minutes.
4. Strain the tea into a cup.
5. Add honey or sweetener if desired.

Nutrition Info (per serving):
- Calories: 0 (without honey or sweetener)
- Protein: 0g
- Fat: 0g
- Carbohydrates: 0g
- Fiber: 0g
- Sodium: 0mg

Servings: 4 **Cooking Time:** 10 minutes

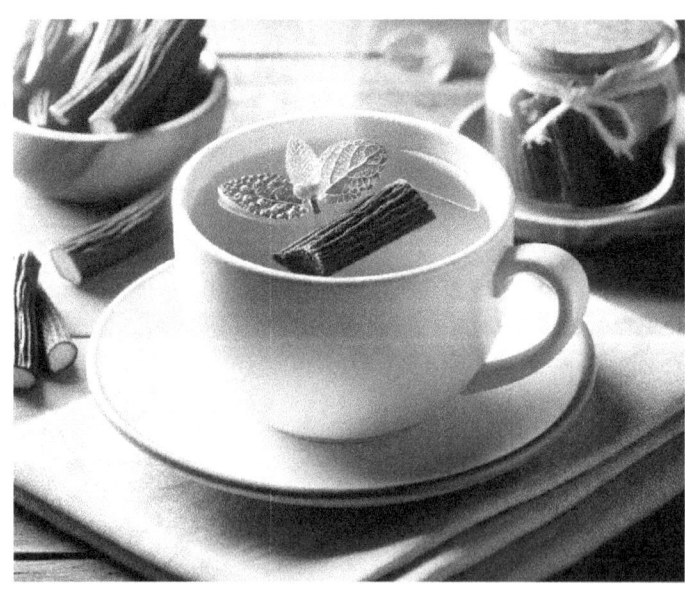

Full Liquid Recipes

1. Smooth Cream of Wheat
Ingredients:
- 1/4 cup Cream of Wheat
- 1 cup low-fat milk or water
- 1/4 teaspoon salt (optional)
- Sweetener (optional)

Instructions:
1. In a saucepan, bring the milk or water and salt to a boil.
2. Gradually stir in the Cream of Wheat.
3. Reduce heat to low and simmer, stirring constantly, for about 2-3 minutes until thickened.
4. Add sweetener if desired.
5. Serve warm.

Nutrition Info (per serving):
- Calories: 120
- Protein: 4g
- Fat: 2g
- Carbohydrates: 23g
- Fiber: 1g
- Sodium: 190mg

Servings: 1 **Cooking Time:** 5 minutes

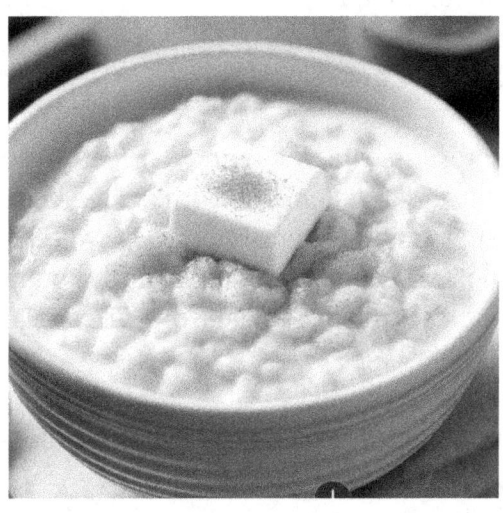

2. Blended Pumpkin Soup

Ingredients:
- 2 cups pumpkin puree (canned or homemade)
- 2 cups low-sodium chicken broth
- 1/2 cup low-fat milk or cream
- 1 small onion, chopped
- 1 garlic clove, minced
- 1/2 teaspoon ground cinnamon
- 1/4 teaspoon ground nutmeg
- Salt and pepper to taste

Instructions:
1. In a large pot, sauté the onion and garlic until soft.
2. Add the pumpkin puree and chicken broth. Stir to combine.
3. Bring to a boil, then reduce heat and simmer for 10 minutes.
4. Stir in the milk or cream, cinnamon, nutmeg, salt, and pepper.
5. Use an immersion blender to blend the soup until smooth.
6. Serve warm.

Nutrition Info (per serving):
Calories: 100 Protein: 2g Fat: 2g Carbohydrates: 18g   Fiber: 4g Sodium: 300mg
Servings: 4 **Cooking Time:** 20 minutes

3. Mashed Potato Soup

Ingredients:
- 2 large potatoes, peeled and diced
- 4 cups low-sodium chicken broth
- 1/2 cup low-fat milk or cream
- 1 small onion, chopped
- 2 garlic cloves, minced
- Salt and pepper to taste

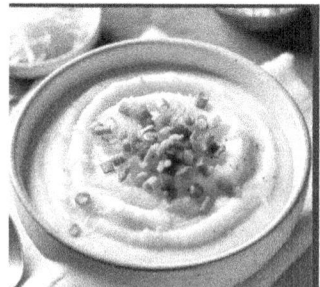

Instructions:
1. In a large pot, sauté the onion and garlic until soft.
2. Add the potatoes and chicken broth. Bring to a boil.
3. Reduce heat and simmer until potatoes are tender, about 15 minutes.
4. Use an immersion blender to blend the soup until smooth.
5. Stir in the milk or cream, and season with salt and pepper.
6. Serve warm.

Nutrition Info (per serving):
- Calories: 120 Protein: 3g Fat: 3g Carbohydrates: 22g
- Fiber: 2g
- Sodium: 300mg

Servings: 4 **Cooking Time:** 25 minutes

4. Pea Soup
Ingredients:
- 2 cups frozen peas
- 2 cups low-sodium vegetable broth
- 1/2 cup low-fat milk or cream
- 1 small onion, chopped
- 2 garlic cloves, minced
- Salt and pepper to taste

Instructions:
1. In a large pot, sauté the onion and garlic until soft.
2. Add the peas and vegetable broth. Bring to a boil.
3. Reduce heat and simmer for 10 minutes.
4. Use an immersion blender to blend the soup until smooth.
5. Stir in the milk or cream, and season with salt and pepper.
6. Serve warm.

Nutrition Info (per serving):
- Calories: 100 Protein: 5g Fat: 2g Carbohydrates: 15g Fiber: 4g
- Sodium: 250mg

Servings: 4 **Cooking Time:** 20 minutes

5. Banana Smoothie
Ingredients:
- 1 ripe banana
- 1 cup low-fat milk or yogurt
- 1/2 cup ice
- 1 teaspoon honey (optional)

Instructions:
1. Combine all ingredients in a blender.
2. Blend until smooth.
3. Serve immediately.

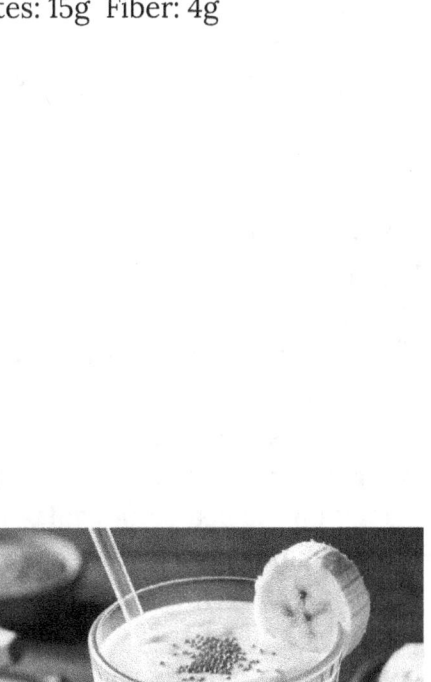

Nutrition Info (per serving):
- Calories: 150
- Protein: 5g
- Fat: 2g
- Carbohydrates: 31g
- Fiber: 2g
- Sodium: 60mg

Servings: 1 **Cooking Time:** 5 minutes

6. Avocado Smoothie

Ingredients:
- 1 ripe avocado
- 1 cup low-fat milk or yogurt
- 1/2 cup ice
- 1 tablespoon honey (optional)
- 1 teaspoon lime juice

Instructions:
1. Combine all ingredients in a blender.
2. Blend until smooth.
3. Serve immediately.

Nutrition Info (per serving):
- Calories: 200
- Protein: 6g
- Fat: 15g
- Carbohydrates: 17g
- Fiber: 7g
- Sodium: 60mg

Servings: 1 **Cooking Time:** 5 minutes

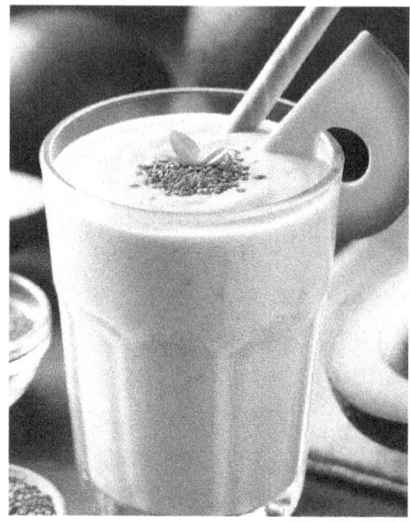

7. Pear & Ricotta Puree

Ingredients:
- 2 ripe pears, peeled and cored
- 1/2 cup ricotta cheese
- 1 tablespoon honey (optional)
- 1/2 teaspoon cinnamon

Instructions:
1. Steam the pears until soft, about 5 minutes.
2. Combine pears, ricotta cheese, honey, and cinnamon in a blender.
3. Blend until smooth.
4. Serve immediately.

Nutrition Info (per serving):
- Calories: 150
- Protein: 5g
- Fat: 4g
- Carbohydrates: 26g
- Fiber: 4g
- Sodium: 40mg

Servings: 2 **Cooking Time:** 10 minutes

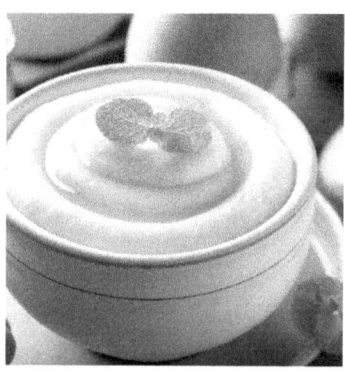

8. Shrimp Scampi Puree
Ingredients:
- 1/2 pound shrimp, peeled and deveined
- 1/2 cup low-sodium chicken broth
- 1/4 cup low-fat cream
- 1 clove garlic, minced
- 1 tablespoon olive oil
- 1 tablespoon lemon juice
- Salt and pepper to taste

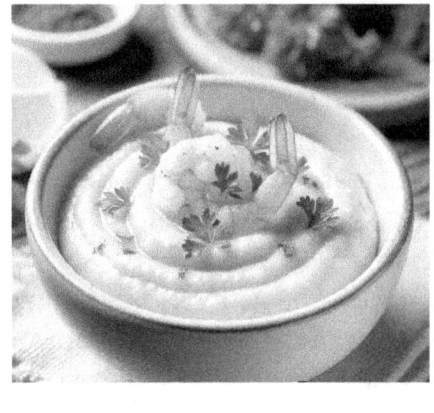

Instructions:
1. In a skillet, heat olive oil over medium heat.
2. Add garlic and sauté until fragrant.
3. Add shrimp and cook until pink, about 3 minutes.
4. Transfer shrimp to a blender.
5. Add chicken broth, cream, lemon juice, salt, and pepper.
6. Blend until smooth.
7. Serve warm.

Nutrition Info (per serving):
- Calories: 120   Protein: 15g Fat: 5g Carbohydrates: 3g
- Fiber: 0g
- Sodium: 200mg

Servings: 2 **Cooking Time:** 10 minutes

9. Yogurt Smoothie
Ingredients:
- 1 cup low-fat yogurt
- 1/2 cup fresh or frozen berries (strawberries, blueberries, raspberries)
- 1/2 cup ice
- 1 tablespoon honey (optional)

Instructions:
1. Combine all ingredients in a blender.
2. Blend until smooth.
3. Serve immediately.

Nutrition Info (per serving):
- Calories: 130
- Protein: 6g
- Fat: 2g
- Carbohydrates: 22g
- Fiber: 2g
- Sodium: 60mg

Servings: 1 **Cooking Time:** 5 minutes

10. Malted Milk Drink

Ingredients:
- 1 cup low-fat milk
- 2 tablespoons malted milk powder
- 1 teaspoon honey (optional)
- 1/4 teaspoon vanilla extract

Instructions:
1. Heat the milk in a saucepan over medium heat until warm, but not boiling.
2. Stir in the malted milk powder until fully dissolved.
3. Add honey and vanilla extract, stirring to combine.
4. Pour into a glass and serve warm.

Nutrition Info (per serving):
- Calories: 150 Protein: 8g Fat: 2.5g Carbohydrates: 24g
- Fiber: 0g
- Sodium: 100mg

Servings: 1 **Cooking Time:** 5 minutes

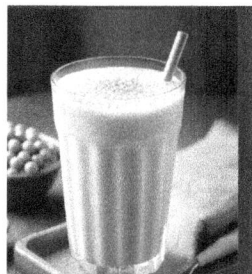

11. Rice Congee

Ingredients:
- 1/2 cup jasmine rice
- 8 cups water or low-sodium chicken broth
- 1-inch piece of ginger, peeled and sliced
- Salt to taste
- Optional toppings: chopped green onions, soy sauce, sesame oil

Instructions:
1. Rinse the rice under cold water until the water runs clear.
2. In a large pot, combine the rice, water or chicken broth, and ginger.
3. Bring to a boil, then reduce heat to low and simmer, stirring occasionally, for 1-1.5 hours until the rice breaks down and the mixture thickens to a porridge-like consistency.
4. Remove the ginger slices and season with salt to taste.
5. Serve warm with optional toppings.

Nutrition Info (per serving):
- Calories: 90
- Protein: 2g
- Fat: 0g
- Carbohydrates: 20g
- Fiber: 0g
- Sodium: 10mg (without additional toppings)

Servings: 6 **Cooking Time:** 1.5 hours

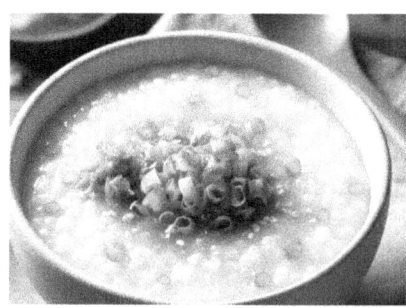

12. Egg Custard

Ingredients:
- 2 large eggs
- 1 cup low-fat milk
- 2 tablespoons sugar
- 1/2 teaspoon vanilla extract
- Pinch of salt

Instructions:
1. Preheat the oven to 350°F (175°C).
2. In a bowl, whisk together the eggs, milk, sugar, vanilla extract, and salt until well combined.
3. Pour the mixture into individual ramekins or a baking dish.
4. Place the ramekins or baking dish in a larger baking pan and fill the pan with hot water halfway up the sides of the ramekins.
5. Bake for 30-35 minutes, or until the custard is set but still slightly jiggly in the center.
6. Remove from the oven and let cool before serving.

Nutrition Info (per serving):
- Calories: 120
- Protein: 7g
- Fat: 4g
- Carbohydrates: 12g
- Fiber: 0g
- Sodium: 90mg

Servings: 4 **Cooking Time:** 45 minutes

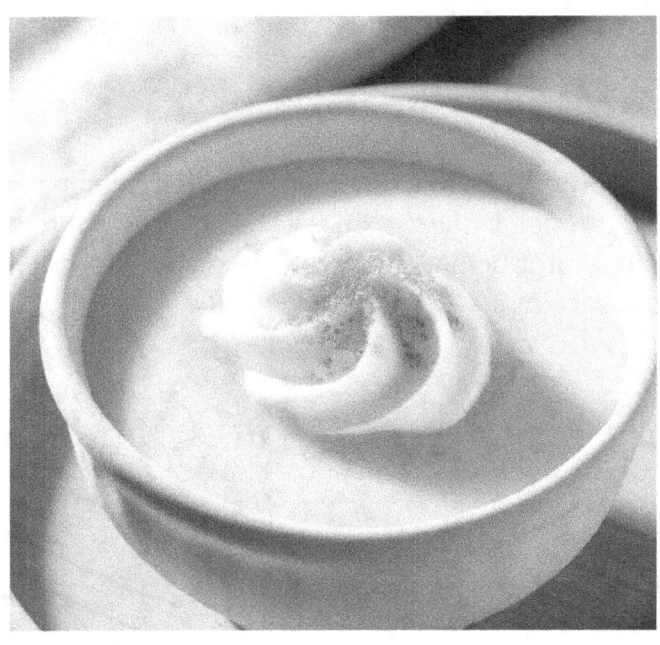

13. Strained Cream Soups

Ingredients:
- 2 cups low-sodium chicken broth or vegetable broth
- 1 cup low-fat milk or cream
- 1 cup cooked vegetables (e.g., carrots, broccoli, cauliflower)
- 1 small onion, chopped
- 1 garlic clove, minced
- Salt and pepper to taste

Instructions:
1. In a large pot, sauté the onion and garlic until soft.
2. Add the cooked vegetables and broth. Bring to a boil.
3. Reduce heat and simmer for 10 minutes.
4. Use an immersion blender to blend the soup until smooth.
5. Stir in the milk or cream and season with salt and pepper.
6. Strain the soup through a fine-mesh sieve to ensure it's completely smooth.
7. Serve warm.

Nutrition Info (per serving):
Calories: 100 Protein: 3g Fat: 3g Carbohydrates: 15g Fiber: 2g
- Sodium: 200mg

Servings: 4 **Cooking Time:** 20 minutes

14. Honeydew Melon Juice

Ingredients:
- 1 ripe honeydew melon, peeled, seeded, and cubed
- 1 tablespoon honey (optional)
- 1/2 cup water (optional, for a thinner consistency)

Instructions:
1. Place the honeydew melon cubes in a blender.
2. Blend until smooth.
3. Add honey and water if desired, blending again until combined.
4. Strain the juice through a fine-mesh sieve or cheesecloth to remove pulp.
5. Chill in the refrigerator before serving.

Nutrition Info (per serving):
- Calories: 50
- Protein: 1g
- Fat: 0g
- Carbohydrates: 13g
- Fiber: 1g
- Sodium: 20mg

Servings: 4 **Cooking Time:** 10 minutes

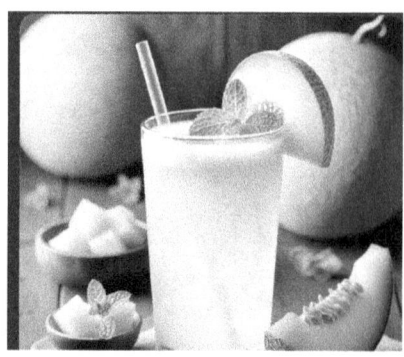

Semisolids/Soft Foods

1. Mashed Sweet Potatoes
Ingredients:
- 2 large sweet potatoes
- 1/4 cup low-fat milk
- 1 tablespoon butter
- Salt and pepper to taste

Instructions:
1. Peel and cube the sweet potatoes.
2. Boil the sweet potatoes in a large pot of water until tender, about 15 minutes.
3. Drain the sweet potatoes and return them to the pot.
4. Add the milk and butter, then mash until smooth.
5. Season with salt and pepper to taste.

Nutrition Info (per serving):
- Calories: 150
- Protein: 2g
- Fat: 4g
- Carbohydrates: 30g
- Fiber: 5g
- Sodium: 50mg

Servings: 4 **Cooking Time:** 20 minutes

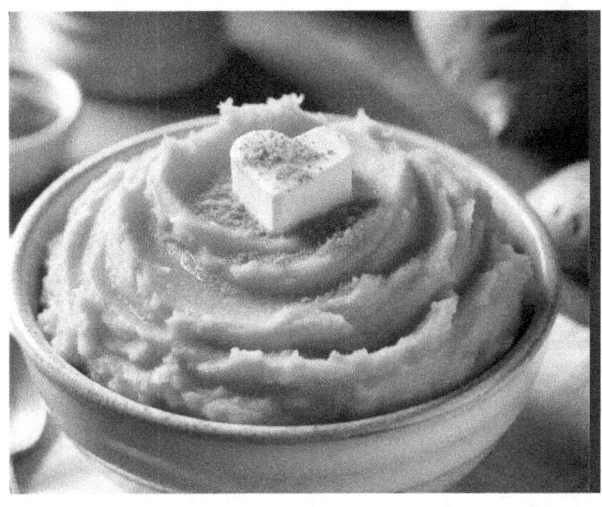

2. Refried Beans

Ingredients:
- 2 cups cooked pinto beans (or one 15-ounce can, drained and rinsed)
- 1 tablespoon olive oil
- 1 small onion, finely chopped
- 1 garlic clove, minced
- 1/2 teaspoon ground cumin
- 1/2 teaspoon chili powder
- Salt to taste

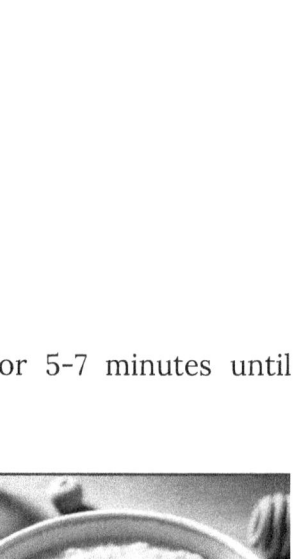

Instructions:
1. Heat the olive oil in a skillet over medium heat.
2. Add the onion and garlic, and sauté until soft.
3. Add the beans, cumin, and chili powder, and cook for 5 minutes.
4. Mash the beans with a potato masher or the back of a spoon until smooth.
5. Season with salt to taste.

Nutrition Info (per serving):
- Calories: 120 Protein: 6g Fat: 4g Carbohydrates: 18g Fiber: 5g
- Sodium: 200mg

Servings: 4 **Cooking Time:** 15 minutes

3. Oatmeal

Ingredients:
- 1 cup rolled oats
- 2 cups water or low-fat milk
- 1/4 teaspoon salt
- Sweetener or fruit toppings (optional)

Instructions:
1. In a pot, bring the water or milk and salt to a boil.
2. Stir in the oats.
3. Reduce heat and simmer, stirring occasionally, for 5-7 minutes until thickened.
4. Add sweetener or fruit toppings if desired.

Nutrition Info (per serving):
- Calories: 150
- Protein: 5g
- Fat: 3g
- Carbohydrates: 27g
- Fiber: 4g
- Sodium: 150mg

Servings: 2 **Cooking Time:** 10 minutes

4. Cream of Rice

Ingredients:
- 1/2 cup cream of rice cereal
- 2 cups water or low-fat milk
- 1/4 teaspoon salt
- Sweetener (optional)

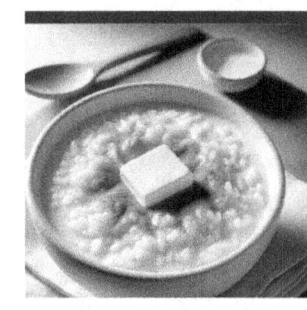

Instructions:
1. In a pot, bring the water or milk and salt to a boil.
2. Gradually stir in the cream of rice.
3. Reduce heat to low and simmer, stirring constantly, for about 3 minutes until thickened.
4. Add sweetener if desired.

Nutrition Info (per serving):
- Calories: 90 Protein: 2g Fat: 0g Carbohydrates: 20g
- Fiber: 0g
- Sodium: 200mg

Servings: 2 **Cooking Time:** 5 minutes

5. Banana Puree

Ingredients:
- 2 ripe bananas

Instructions:
1. Peel and slice the bananas.
2. Place the bananas in a blender or food processor.
3. Blend until smooth.
4. Serve immediately.

Nutrition Info (per serving):
- Calories: 90
- Protein: 1g
- Fat: 0g
- Carbohydrates: 23g
- Fiber: 2g
- Sodium: 0mg

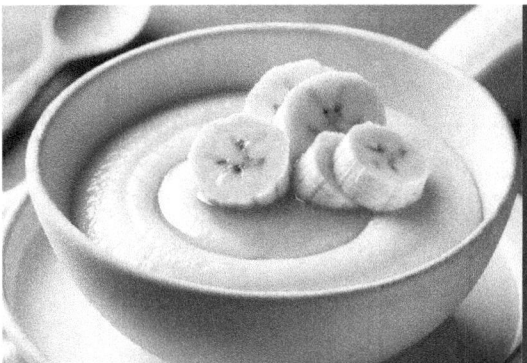

Servings: 2 **Cooking Time:** 5 minutes

6. Fluffy Egg Whites

Ingredients:
- 4 large egg whites
- 1 tablespoon low-fat milk
- Salt and pepper to taste
- Non-stick cooking spray

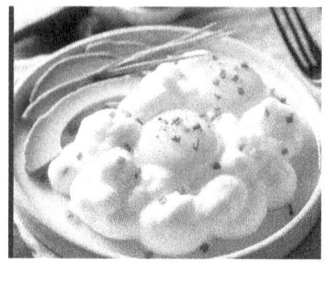

Instructions:
1. In a bowl, whisk the egg whites and milk until frothy.
2. Spray a non-stick skillet with cooking spray and heat over medium heat.
3. Pour the egg white mixture into the skillet.
4. Cook, stirring gently, until the egg whites are set and fluffy, about 3-4 minutes.
5. Season with salt and pepper to taste.

Nutrition Info (per serving):
- Calories: 60
- Protein: 12g
- Fat: 0g
- Carbohydrates: 1g
- Fiber: 0g
- Sodium: 150mg

Servings: 2 **Cooking Time:** 5 minutes

7. Soft Cheesecake

Ingredients:
- 8 ounces low-fat cream cheese, softened
- 1/2 cup Greek yogurt
- 1/4 cup honey or sweetener
- 1 teaspoon vanilla extract

Instructions:
1. In a bowl, beat the cream cheese until smooth.
2. Add the Greek yogurt, honey, and vanilla extract, and mix until well combined.
3. Divide the mixture into small ramekins.
4. Chill in the refrigerator for at least 2 hours before serving.

Nutrition Info (per serving):
- Calories: 120
- Protein: 6g
- Fat: 5g
- Carbohydrates: 14g
- Fiber: 0g
- Sodium: 180mg

Servings: 4 **Cooking Time:** 2 hours (chilling time)

8. Baba Ghanoush

Ingredients:
- 1 large eggplant
- 1/4 cup tahini
- 2 tablespoons lemon juice
- 2 garlic cloves, minced
- Salt to taste
- Olive oil for drizzling

Instructions:
1. Preheat the oven to 400°F (200°C).
2. Prick the eggplant with a fork and place on a baking sheet.
3. Roast the eggplant for 30-40 minutes, until soft.
4. Allow the eggplant to cool, then peel and scoop out the flesh.
5. In a food processor, combine the eggplant, tahini, lemon juice, garlic, and salt.
6. Blend until smooth.
7. Drizzle with olive oil before serving.

Nutrition Info (per serving):
- Calories: 80 Protein: 2g Fat: 6g Carbohydrates: 7g Fiber: 3g
- Sodium: 150mg

Servings: 4 **Cooking Time:** 45 minutes

9. Protein Pancakes

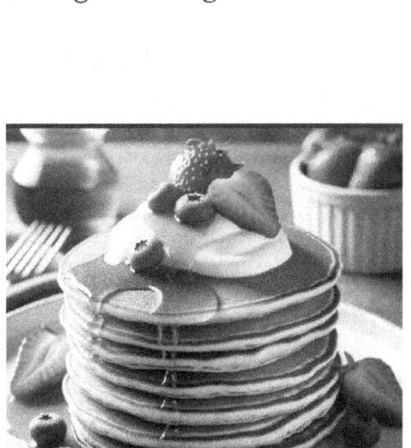

Ingredients:
- 1/2 cup rolled oats
- 1/2 cup low-fat cottage cheese
- 1/4 cup egg whites
- 1/2 teaspoon baking powder
- 1 teaspoon vanilla extract
- Non-stick cooking spray

Instructions:
1. Blend all ingredients in a blender until smooth.
2. Spray a non-stick skillet with cooking spray and heat over medium heat.
3. Pour the batter into the skillet to form pancakes.
4. Cook until bubbles form on the surface, then flip and cook until golden brown, about 2-3 minutes per side.
5. Serve warm.

Nutrition Info (per serving):
- Calories: 180 Protein: 15g Fat: 3g Carbohydrates: 23g
- Fiber: 3g
- Sodium: 200mg

Servings: 2 **Cooking Time:** 10 minutes

10. Corned Beef

Ingredients:
- 1 pound corned beef
- 1 small onion, chopped
- 2 garlic cloves, minced
- 2 cups water

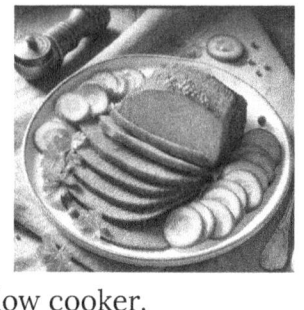

Instructions:
1. Place the corned beef, onion, garlic, and water in a slow cooker.
2. Cook on low for 8 hours, or until the beef is tender.
3. Shred the beef with a fork before serving.

Nutrition Info (per serving):
- Calories: 250 Protein: 18g Fat: 18g
- Carbohydrates: 1g
- Fiber: 0g
- Sodium: 800mg

Servings: 4 **Cooking Time:** 8 hours

11. Apple Crumbled Ramekins

Ingredients:
- 2 large apples, peeled, cored, and chopped
- 1/4 cup rolled oats
- 2 tablespoons whole wheat flour
- 2 tablespoons brown sugar
- 2 tablespoons cold butter, cubed
- 1/2 teaspoon cinnamon

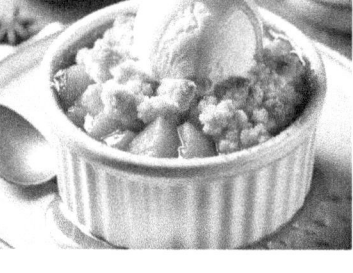

Instructions:
1. Preheat the oven to 350°F (175°C).
2. Divide the chopped apples among four ramekins.
3. In a bowl, combine the oats, flour, brown sugar, and cinnamon.
4. Cut in the butter until the mixture resembles coarse crumbs.
5. Sprinkle the oat mixture over the apples.
6. Bake for 20-25 minutes, until the topping is golden brown.

Nutrition Info (per serving):
- Calories: 150
- Protein: 2g
- Fat: 6g
- Carbohydrates: 25g
- Fiber: 3g
- Sodium: 50mg

Servings: 4 **Cooking Time:** 25 minutes

12. Patty Pan Squash

Ingredients:
- 4 small patty pan squashes, halved
- 2 tablespoons olive oil
- 1 garlic clove, minced
- Salt and pepper to taste
- Fresh parsley for garnish (optional)

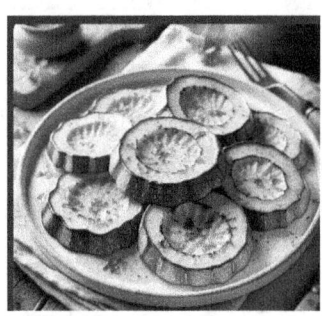

Instructions:
1. Preheat the oven to 400°F (200°C).
2. Toss the squash halves with olive oil, garlic, salt, and pepper.
3. Place the squash on a baking sheet.
4. Roast for 20 minutes, until tender.
5. Garnish with fresh parsley before serving.

Nutrition Info (per serving):
- Calories: 70   Protein: 1g   Fat: 7g   Carbohydrates: 4g   Fiber: 2g
- Sodium: 150mg

Servings: 4 **Cooking Time:** 20 minutes

13. Queso Chicken

Ingredients:
- 1 pound boneless, skinless chicken breasts
- 1 cup salsa
- 1/2 cup shredded low-fat cheddar cheese
- 1/4 cup low-fat cream cheese
- 1 teaspoon taco seasoning

Instructions:
1. Preheat the oven to 375°F (190°C).
2. Place the chicken breasts in a baking dish.
3. Spread the salsa over the chicken.
4. Bake for 25-30 minutes, until the chicken is cooked through.
5. In a small bowl, combine the cheddar cheese, cream cheese, and taco seasoning.
6. Spread the cheese mixture over the chicken and bake for an additional 5 minutes, until the cheese is melted and bubbly.
7. Serve warm.

Nutrition Info (per serving):
- Calories: 220   Protein: 28g   Fat: 9g   Carbohydrates: 5g
- Fiber: 1g
- Sodium: 600mg

Servings: 4 **Cooking Time:** 35 minutes

14. Savory Quinoa Muffins

Ingredients:
- 1 cup cooked quinoa
- 1/2 cup grated zucchini
- 1/4 cup grated carrot
- 1/4 cup finely chopped spinach
- 1/4 cup grated low-fat cheddar cheese
- 2 large eggs
- 1/4 cup low-fat milk
- 1/4 teaspoon salt
- 1/4 teaspoon black pepper
- 1/2 teaspoon baking powder

Instructions:
1. Preheat the oven to 350°F (175°C).
2. In a large bowl, combine the cooked quinoa, grated zucchini, grated carrot, chopped spinach, and grated cheddar cheese.
3. In a separate bowl, whisk together the eggs, milk, salt, black pepper, and baking powder.
4. Pour the egg mixture into the quinoa mixture and stir until well combined.
5. Grease a muffin tin with non-stick cooking spray and divide the mixture evenly among the muffin cups.
6. Bake for 20-25 minutes, or until the muffins are set and lightly golden.
7. Allow the muffins to cool slightly before serving.

Nutrition Info (per serving):
- Calories: 80
- Protein: 5g
- Fat: 3g
- Carbohydrates: 8g
- Fiber: 1g
- Sodium: 150mg

Servings: 12 muffins **Cooking Time:** 30 minutes

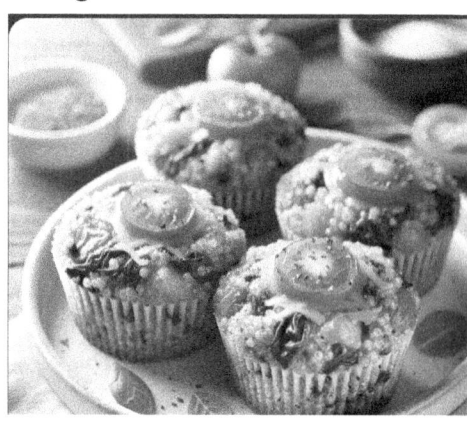

15. Greek Turkey Burgers

Ingredients:
- 1 pound ground turkey
- 1/4 cup crumbled feta cheese
- 1/4 cup finely chopped spinach
- 1/4 cup finely chopped red onion
- 1 garlic clove, minced
- 1 teaspoon dried oregano
- 1/2 teaspoon salt
- 1/4 teaspoon black pepper
- Non-stick cooking spray

Instructions:
1. In a large bowl, combine the ground turkey, feta cheese, spinach, red onion, garlic, oregano, salt, and black pepper.
2. Mix until well combined.
3. Shape the mixture into 4 patties.
4. Spray a non-stick skillet with cooking spray and heat over medium-high heat.
5. Cook the patties for 5-6 minutes per side, or until fully cooked through and no longer pink in the center.
6. Serve warm.

Nutrition Info (per serving):
- Calories: 180 Protein: 25g Fat: 8g Carbohydrates: 2g Fiber: 0g
- Sodium: 400mg

Servings: 4 **Cooking Time:** 15 minutes

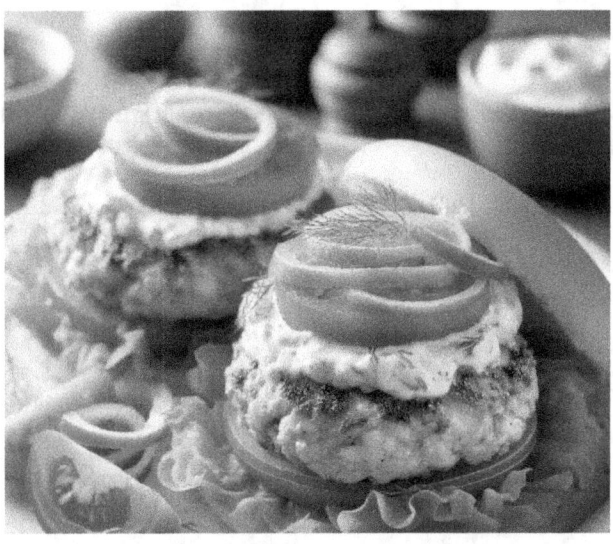

16. Ruby French Dressing

Ingredients:
- 1/2 cup ketchup
- 1/4 cup white vinegar
- 1/4 cup olive oil
- 1/4 cup finely chopped onion
- 2 tablespoons honey
- 1 tablespoon lemon juice
- 1 teaspoon Worcestershire sauce
- 1/2 teaspoon paprika
- 1/4 teaspoon salt
- 1/4 teaspoon black pepper

Instructions:
1. In a blender or food processor, combine the ketchup, white vinegar, olive oil, chopped onion, honey, lemon juice, Worcestershire sauce, paprika, salt, and black pepper.
2. Blend until smooth and well combined.
3. Transfer the dressing to a jar or container with a lid.
4. Refrigerate for at least 1 hour before serving to allow the flavors to meld together.

Nutrition Info (per serving):
- Calories: 80
- Protein: 0g
- Fat: 7g
- Carbohydrates: 5g
- Fiber: 0g
- Sodium: 200mg

Servings: 8 (2 tablespoons per serving) **Cooking Time:** 5 minutes (plus 1 hour refrigeration time)

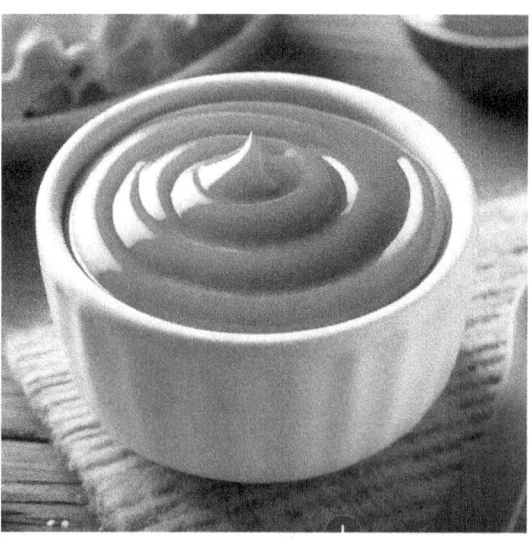

Breakfast Recipes

1. Greek Yogurt with Mashed Berries
Ingredients:
- 1 cup plain Greek yogurt
- 1/2 cup mixed berries (strawberries, blueberries, raspberries)
- 1 teaspoon honey or agave syrup (optional)

Instructions:
1. In a small bowl, mash the berries with a fork until they reach your desired consistency.
2. In a serving bowl, combine the Greek yogurt and mashed berries.
3. Drizzle with honey or agave syrup if desired.
4. Serve immediately.

Nutrition Info (per serving):
- Calories: 150
- Protein: 14g
- Fat: 4g
- Carbohydrates: 16g
- Fiber: 3g
- Sodium: 60mg

Servings: 1 **Cooking Time:** 5 minutes

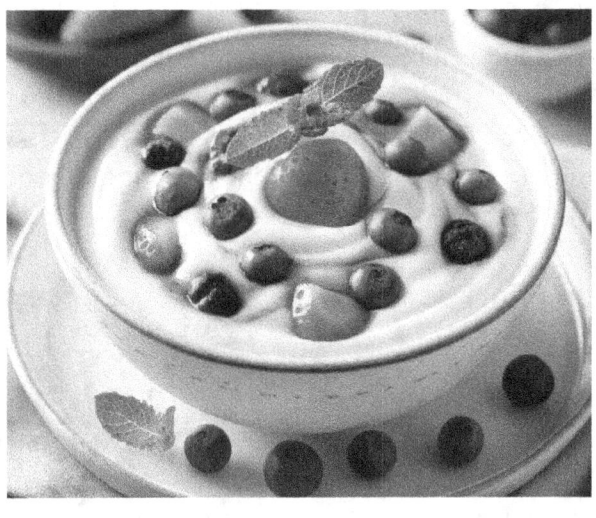

2. Protein Powder Porridge

Ingredients:
- 1/2 cup rolled oats
- 1 cup water or low-fat milk
- 1 scoop protein powder (vanilla or unflavored)
- 1/2 teaspoon cinnamon

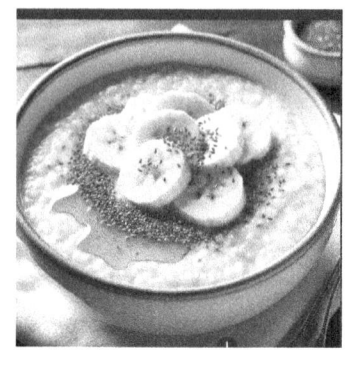

Instructions:
1. In a pot, bring the water or milk to a boil.
2. Stir in the oats and reduce heat to a simmer.
3. Cook for 5-7 minutes, stirring occasionally, until thickened.
4. Remove from heat and stir in the protein powder and cinnamon.
5. Serve warm.

Nutrition Info (per serving):
- Calories: 220 Protein: 20g Fat: 4g Carbohydrates: 30g Fiber: 4g
- Sodium: 150mg

Servings: 1 **Cooking Time:** 10 minutes

3. Silken Tofu Scramble

Ingredients:
- 1 block silken tofu
- 1/2 cup diced tomatoes
- 1/4 cup chopped spinach
- 1/4 teaspoon turmeric
- 1/4 teaspoon garlic powder
- 1/4 teaspoon onion powder

Instructions:
1. Heat a non-stick skillet over medium heat.
2. Add the silken tofu and break it up with a spatula.
3. Add the diced tomatoes and chopped spinach.
4. Sprinkle with turmeric, garlic powder, and onion powder.
5. Cook for 5-7 minutes, stirring occasionally, until heated through and the spinach is wilted.
6. Serve warm.

Nutrition Info (per serving):
- Calories: 120
- Protein: 10g
- Fat: 6g
- Carbohydrates: 8g
- Fiber: 2g
- Sodium: 100mg

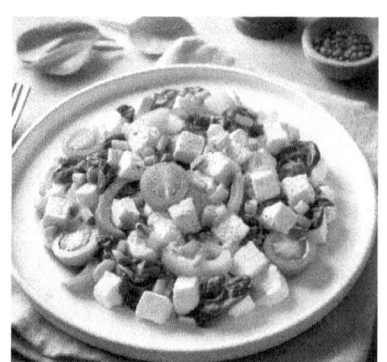

Servings: 2 **Cooking Time:** 10 minutes

4. Savory Mashed Pumpkin

Ingredients:
- 1 cup pumpkin puree
- 1 tablespoon low-fat cream cheese
- 1/4 teaspoon ground nutmeg
- 1/4 teaspoon cinnamon

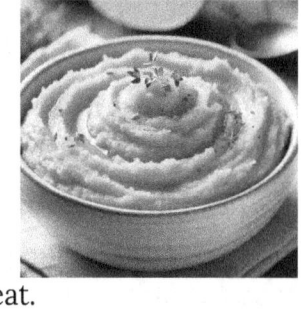

Instructions:
1. In a saucepan, heat the pumpkin puree over medium heat.
2. Stir in the low-fat cream cheese until melted and well combined.
3. Add the ground nutmeg and cinnamon, stirring to combine.
4. Serve warm.

Nutrition Info (per serving):
- Calories: 100 Protein: 3g Fat: 2g Carbohydrates: 19g Fiber: 5g
- Sodium: 30mg

Servings: 2 **Cooking Time:** 5 minutes

5. Creamed Barley

Ingredients:
- 1/2 cup pearl barley
- 2 cups water
- 1/2 cup low-fat milk
- 1 tablespoon honey
- 1/2 teaspoon vanilla extract

Instructions:
1. In a pot, bring the water to a boil.
2. Add the barley and reduce heat to a simmer.
3. Cook for 30-40 minutes, until the barley is tender.
4. Drain any excess water.
5. Return the barley to the pot and stir in the milk, honey, and vanilla extract.
6. Cook for an additional 5 minutes, stirring frequently, until creamy.
7. Serve warm.

Nutrition Info (per serving):
- Calories: 150
- Protein: 4g
- Fat: 1g
- Carbohydrates: 32g
- Fiber: 6g
- Sodium: 30mg

Servings: 3 **Cooking Time:** 45 minutes

6. Vegetable Juice Smoothie

Ingredients:
- 1 cup carrot juice
- 1/2 cup spinach
- 1/2 cucumber, peeled and chopped
- 1/2 apple, cored and chopped
- 1 teaspoon lemon juice

Instructions:
1. Place all ingredients in a blender.
2. Blend until smooth.
3. Serve immediately.

Nutrition Info (per serving):
- Calories: 90
- Protein: 2g
- Fat: 0g
- Carbohydrates: 22g
- Fiber: 3g
- Sodium: 60mg

Servings: 1 **Cooking Time:** 5 minutes

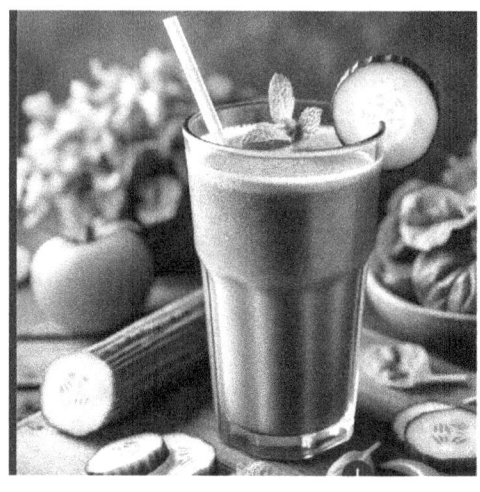

7. Kefir with Pureed Mango

Ingredients:
- 1 cup plain kefir
- 1/2 cup fresh or frozen mango, diced
- 1 teaspoon honey (optional)

Instructions:
1. In a blender, puree the diced mango until smooth.
2. In a serving bowl, combine the kefir and pureed mango.
3. Drizzle with honey if desired.
4. Serve immediately.

Nutrition Info (per serving):
- Calories: 140
- Protein: 6g
- Fat: 2g
- Carbohydrates: 26g
- Fiber: 2g
- Sodium: 60mg

Servings: 1 **Cooking Time:** 5 minutes

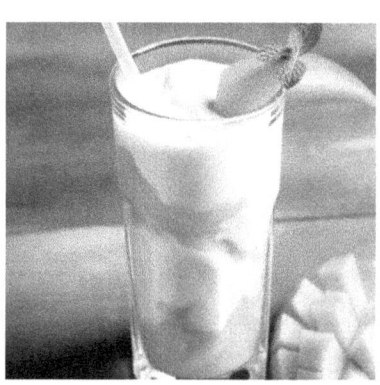

8. Low-fat Quark Cheese

Ingredients:
- 1 cup low-fat quark cheese
- 1 tablespoon honey
- 1/2 teaspoon vanilla extract
- 1/4 cup fresh berries (optional)

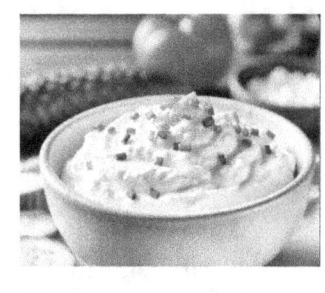

Instructions:
1. In a bowl, mix the quark cheese, honey, and vanilla extract until well combined.
2. Top with fresh berries if desired.
3. Serve immediately.

Nutrition Info (per serving):
- Calories: 120 Protein: 10g Fat: 3g Carbohydrates: 14g Fiber: 1g
- Sodium: 40mg

Servings: 1 **Cooking Time:** 5 minutes

9. Butternut Squash and Apple Mash

Ingredients:
- 1 cup cooked butternut squash, mashed
- 1/2 cup unsweetened applesauce
- 1/4 teaspoon ground cinnamon
- 1/4 teaspoon ground ginger

Instructions:
1. In a bowl, combine the mashed butternut squash and unsweetened applesauce.
2. Stir in the ground cinnamon and ground ginger.
3. Serve warm.

Nutrition Info (per serving):
- Calories: 90
- Protein: 1g
- Fat: 0g
- Carbohydrates: 22g
- Fiber: 4g
- Sodium: 20mg

Servings: 2 **Cooking Time:** 5 minutes

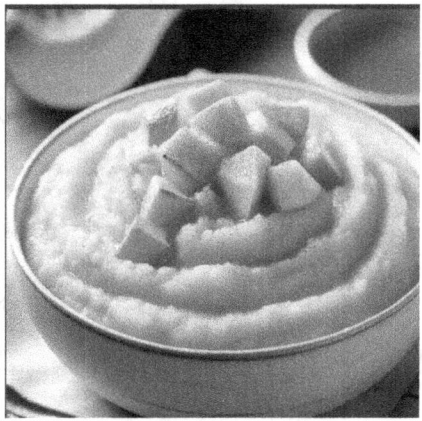

10. Carrot and Zucchini Bread Pudding

Ingredients:
- 1 cup grated carrot
- 1 cup grated zucchini
- 2 slices whole wheat bread, cubed
- 2 large eggs
- 1 cup low-fat milk
- 1/4 cup grated low-fat cheddar cheese
- 1/4 teaspoon ground nutmeg

Instructions:
1. Preheat the oven to 350°F (175°C).
2. In a bowl, combine the grated carrot, grated zucchini, and bread cubes.
3. In a separate bowl, whisk together the eggs, milk, grated cheese, and ground nutmeg.
4. Pour the egg mixture over the vegetable and bread mixture, stirring to combine.
5. Pour the mixture into a greased baking dish.
6. Bake for 30-35 minutes, or until the pudding is set and lightly golden.
7. Allow to cool slightly before serving.

Nutrition Info (per serving):
- Calories: 180
- Protein: 10g
- Fat: 6g
- Carbohydrates: 20g
- Fiber: 3g
- Sodium: 200mg

Servings: 4 **Cooking Time:** 35 minutes

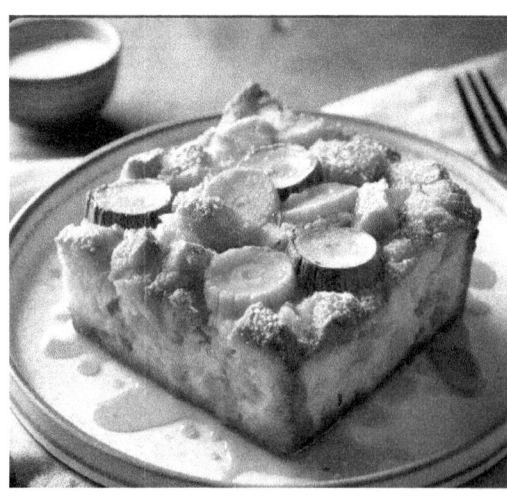

11. Protein Enriched Apple Smoothie
Ingredients:
- 1 medium apple, peeled and chopped
- 1 cup unsweetened almond milk
- 1 scoop vanilla protein powder
- 1/2 teaspoon ground cinnamon
- 1/2 cup ice cubes

Instructions:
1. Place all ingredients in a blender.
2. Blend until smooth.
3. Serve immediately.

Nutrition Info (per serving):
- Calories: 200
- Protein: 20g
- Fat: 3g
- Carbohydrates: 28g
- Fiber: 4g
- Sodium: 150mg

Servings: 1 **Cooking Time:** 5 minutes

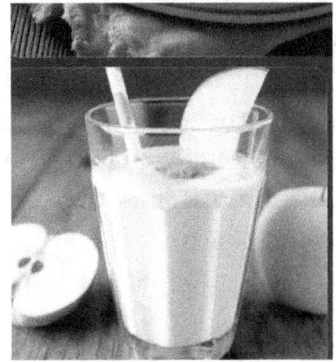

12. Steamed Vegetable Puree
Ingredients:
- 1 cup broccoli florets
- 1 cup cauliflower florets
- 1 small carrot, peeled and sliced
- 1/4 cup low-sodium vegetable broth

Instructions:
1. Steam the broccoli, cauliflower, and carrot until tender, about 10 minutes.
2. Place the steamed vegetables in a blender or food processor.
3. Add the vegetable broth and blend until smooth.
4. Serve warm.

Nutrition Info (per serving):
- Calories: 60
- Protein: 3g
- Fat: 0g
- Carbohydrates: 12g
- Fiber: 5g
- Sodium: 100mg

Servings: 2 **Cooking Time:** 15 minutes

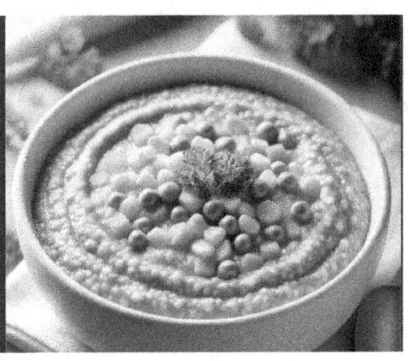

13. Sweet Potato Puree

Ingredients:
- 2 medium sweet potatoes, peeled and cubed
- 1/4 cup low-fat milk
- 1 tablespoon maple syrup
- 1/2 teaspoon ground cinnamon

Instructions:
1. Boil the sweet potatoes in a pot of water until tender, about 15 minutes.
2. Drain the sweet potatoes and place them in a blender or food processor.
3. Add the milk, maple syrup, and cinnamon.
4. Blend until smooth.
5. Serve warm.

Nutrition Info (per serving):
- Calories: 120 Protein: 2g Fat: 1g Carbohydrates: 28g Fiber: 4g
- Sodium: 40mg

Servings: 2 **Cooking Time:** 20 minutes

14. Soy Yogurt Parfait

Ingredients:
- 1 cup plain soy yogurt
- 1/4 cup granola (low-fat)
- 1/2 cup mixed berries (strawberries, blueberries, raspberries)
- 1 teaspoon honey (optional)

Instructions:
1. In a serving bowl or glass, layer half of the soy yogurt.
2. Add a layer of half the granola and half the mixed berries.
3. Repeat the layers with the remaining yogurt, granola, and berries.
4. Drizzle with honey if desired.
5. Serve immediately.

Nutrition Info (per serving):
- Calories: 220
- Protein: 6g
- Fat: 7g
- Carbohydrates: 34g
- Fiber: 5g
- Sodium: 80mg

Servings: 1 **Cooking Time:** 5 minutes

15. Acorn Squash Puree

Ingredients:
- 1 medium acorn squash, halved and seeded
- 1/4 cup low-sodium chicken broth
- 1 tablespoon maple syrup
- 1/4 teaspoon ground nutmeg

Instructions:
1. Preheat the oven to 375°F (190°C).
2. Place the acorn squash halves on a baking sheet, cut side down.
3. Roast for 40-45 minutes, until tender.
4. Scoop out the flesh of the squash and place it in a blender or food processor.
5. Add the chicken broth, maple syrup, and nutmeg.
6. Blend until smooth.
7. Serve warm.

Nutrition Info (per serving):
- Calories: 100
- Protein: 2g
- Fat: 0g
- Carbohydrates: 26g
- Fiber: 3g
- Sodium: 100mg

Servings: 2 **Cooking Time:** 50 minutes

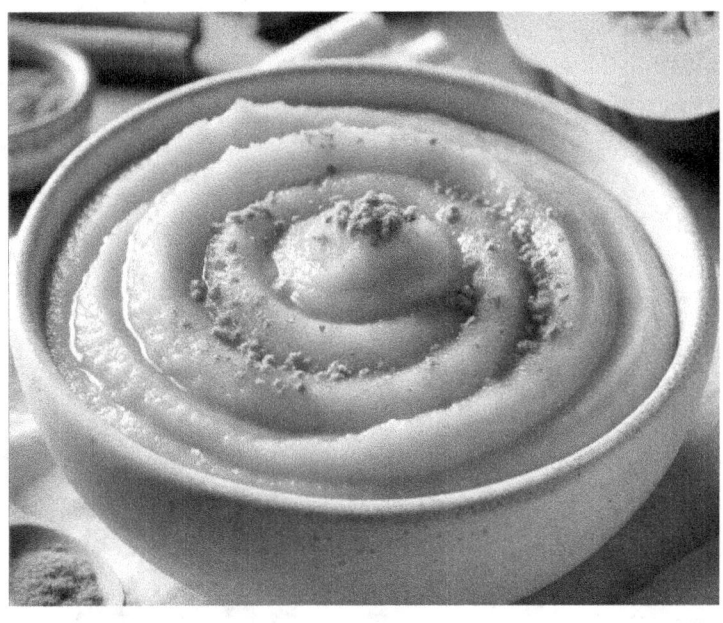

16. Soft Papaya Mash

Ingredients:
- 1 ripe papaya, peeled, seeded, and cubed
- 1 tablespoon lime juice
- 1 teaspoon honey (optional)

Instructions:
1. Place the papaya cubes in a blender or food processor.
2. Add the lime juice and honey if desired.
3. Blend until smooth.
4. Serve immediately.

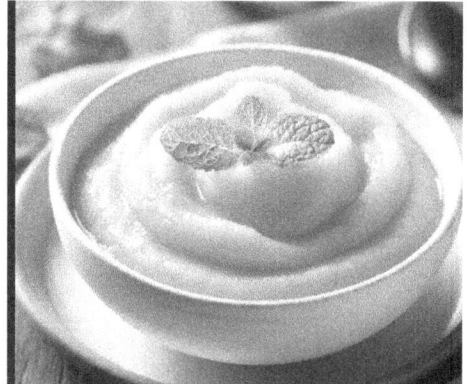

Nutrition Info (per serving):
- Calories: 90
- Protein: 1g
- Fat: 0g
- Carbohydrates: 24g
- Fiber: 3g
- Sodium: 5mg

Servings: 2 **Cooking Time:** 5 minutes

17. Low-fat Milk Porridge

Ingredients:
- 1/2 cup rolled oats
- 1 cup low-fat milk
- 1/4 teaspoon ground cinnamon
- 1 teaspoon honey (optional)

Instructions:
1. In a pot, combine the rolled oats and low-fat milk.
2. Bring to a boil, then reduce heat and simmer, stirring occasionally, for 5-7 minutes until thickened.
3. Stir in the ground cinnamon.
4. Drizzle with honey if desired.
5. Serve warm.

Nutrition Info (per serving):
- Calories: 150
- Protein: 6g
- Fat: 3g
- Carbohydrates: 25g
- Fiber: 3g
- Sodium: 60mg

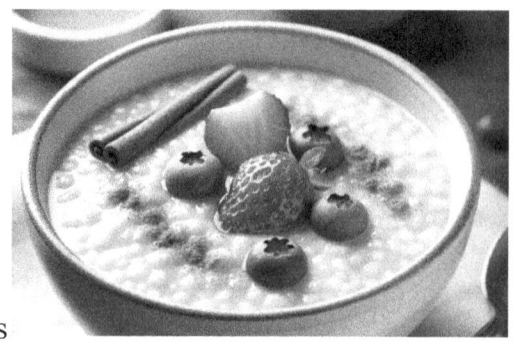

Servings: 1 **Cooking Time:** 10 minutes

18. Liquidized Porridge Pancakes

Ingredients:
- 1/2 cup rolled oats
- 1/2 cup low-fat milk
- 1 large egg
- 1/2 teaspoon baking powder
- 1/2 teaspoon vanilla extract
- Non-stick cooking spray

Instructions:
1. Place the rolled oats in a blender and blend until they become a fine powder.
2. In a bowl, combine the oat powder, low-fat milk, egg, baking powder, and vanilla extract.
3. Blend until smooth.
4. Heat a non-stick skillet over medium heat and spray with cooking spray.
5. Pour small amounts of the batter into the skillet to form pancakes.
6. Cook until bubbles form on the surface, then flip and cook until golden brown, about 2-3 minutes per side.
7. Serve warm.

Nutrition Info (per serving):
- Calories: 180
- Protein: 9g
- Fat: 5g
- Carbohydrates: 24g
- Fiber: 3g
- Sodium: 150mg

Servings: 2 **Cooking Time:** 10 minutes

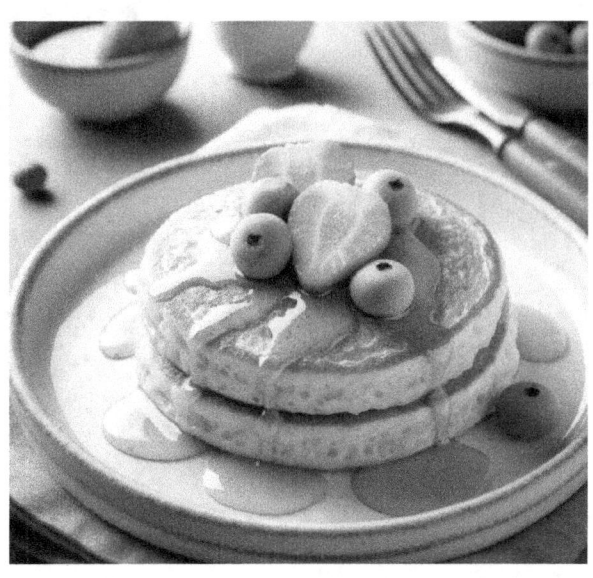

Poultry & Meat

1. Ground Turkey Soup
Ingredients:
- 1 pound ground turkey
- 1 small onion, chopped
- 2 garlic cloves, minced
- 1 cup chopped carrots
- 1 cup chopped celery
- 1 cup diced tomatoes (canned, with juice)
- 4 cups low-sodium chicken broth
- 1 teaspoon dried thyme
- 1 teaspoon dried basil
- 1 cup chopped spinach

Instructions:
1. In a large pot, cook the ground turkey over medium heat until browned, breaking it up with a spoon.
2. Add the chopped onion and garlic, and sauté until softened, about 5 minutes.
3. Add the carrots, celery, diced tomatoes, chicken broth, thyme, and basil.
4. Bring to a boil, then reduce heat and simmer for 20 minutes.
5. Stir in the chopped spinach and cook for an additional 5 minutes.
6. Serve warm.

Nutrition Info (per serving):
- Calories: 180
- Protein: 20g
- Fat: 6g
- Carbohydrates: 12g
- Fiber: 3g
- Sodium: 150mg

Servings: 4 **Cooking Time:** 35 minutes

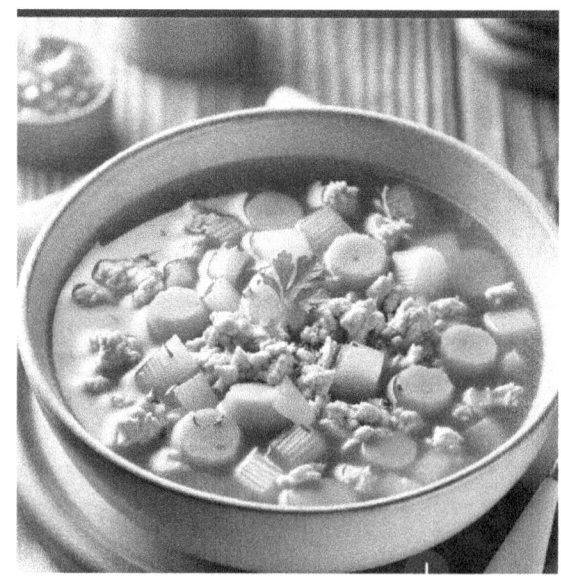

2. Soft Cooked Chicken Thighs

Ingredients:
- 4 boneless, skinless chicken thighs
- 1 cup low-sodium chicken broth
- 1 tablespoon olive oil
- 1 teaspoon dried oregano
- 1 teaspoon garlic powder
- 1/2 teaspoon paprika

Instructions:
1. Preheat the oven to 375°F (190°C).
2. In a small bowl, mix the olive oil, oregano, garlic powder, and paprika.
3. Rub the mixture over the chicken thighs.
4. Place the chicken thighs in a baking dish and pour the chicken broth over them.
5. Cover with foil and bake for 30 minutes, until the chicken is tender and cooked through.
6. Serve warm.

Nutrition Info (per serving):
- Calories: 200
- Protein: 25g
- Fat: 10g
- Carbohydrates: 1g
- Fiber: 0g
- Sodium: 120mg

Servings: 4 **Cooking Time:** 35 minutes

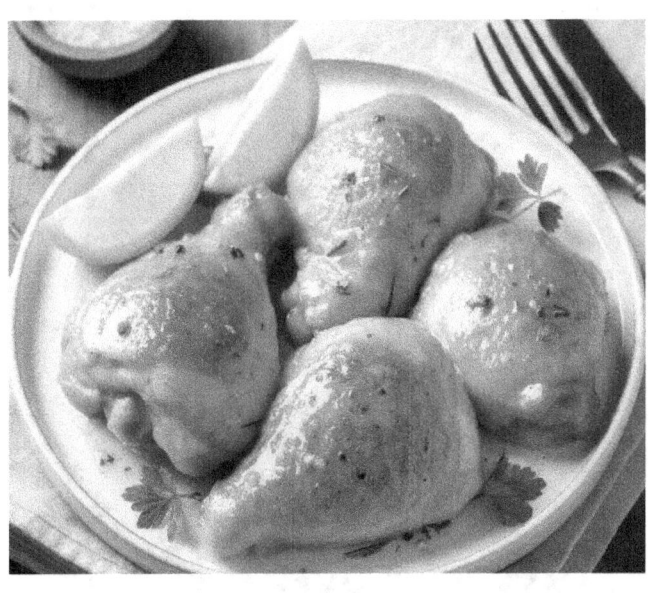

3. Pulled Pork

Ingredients:
- 2 pounds pork shoulder
- 1 cup low-sodium chicken broth
- 1/2 cup apple cider vinegar
- 1/4 cup low-sugar BBQ sauce
- 1 tablespoon smoked paprika
- 1 tablespoon garlic powder
- 1 teaspoon onion powder

Instructions:
1. Place the pork shoulder in a slow cooker.
2. In a small bowl, mix the chicken broth, apple cider vinegar, BBQ sauce, smoked paprika, garlic powder, and onion powder.
3. Pour the mixture over the pork.
4. Cook on low for 8 hours, until the pork is tender and easily shredded with a fork.
5. Remove the pork from the slow cooker and shred with two forks.
6. Return the shredded pork to the slow cooker and mix with the juices.
7. Serve warm.

Nutrition Info (per serving):
- Calories: 250
- Protein: 24g
- Fat: 14g
- Carbohydrates: 4g
- Fiber: 0g
- Sodium: 200mg

Servings: 6 **Cooking Time:** 8 hours

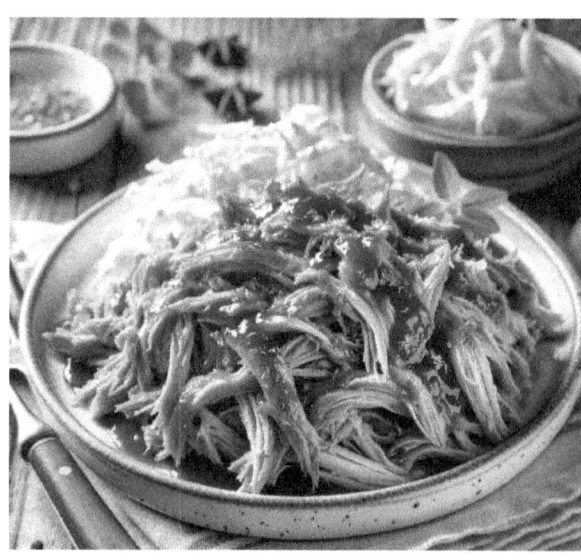

4. Beef Tenderloin Puree

Ingredients:
- 1 pound beef tenderloin, trimmed and cubed
- 1 small onion, chopped
- 1 garlic clove, minced
- 2 cups low-sodium beef broth
- 1/2 teaspoon dried thyme
- 1/2 teaspoon dried rosemary

Instructions:
1. In a large pot, heat a small amount of oil over medium heat.
2. Add the beef tenderloin cubes and cook until browned on all sides.
3. Add the chopped onion and garlic, and sauté until softened, about 5 minutes.
4. Pour in the beef broth, thyme, and rosemary.
5. Bring to a boil, then reduce heat and simmer for 30 minutes, until the beef is very tender.
6. Use an immersion blender to puree the mixture until smooth.
7. Serve warm.

Nutrition Info (per serving):
- Calories: 220
- Protein: 28g
- Fat: 10g
- Carbohydrates: 4g
- Fiber: 1g
- Sodium: 150mg

Servings: 4 **Cooking Time:** 45 minutes

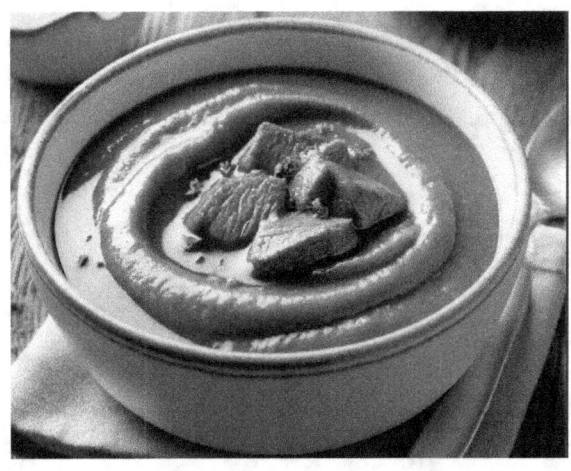

5. Pork Tenderloin Mousse

Ingredients:
- 1 pound pork tenderloin, trimmed and cubed
- 1 small onion, chopped
- 1 garlic clove, minced
- 1/2 cup low-sodium chicken broth
- 1/4 cup low-fat cream cheese
- 1 teaspoon dried sage

Instructions:
1. In a large pot, heat a small amount of oil over medium heat.
2. Add the pork tenderloin cubes and cook until browned on all sides.
3. Add the chopped onion and garlic, and sauté until softened, about 5 minutes.
4. Pour in the chicken broth and sage.
5. Bring to a boil, then reduce heat and simmer for 20 minutes, until the pork is very tender.
6. Transfer the mixture to a blender and add the cream cheese.
7. Blend until smooth and creamy.
8. Serve warm.

Nutrition Info (per serving):
- Calories: 180
- Protein: 24g
- Fat: 7g
- Carbohydrates: 3g
- Fiber: 0g
- Sodium: 130mg

Servings: 4 **Cooking Time:** 30 minutes

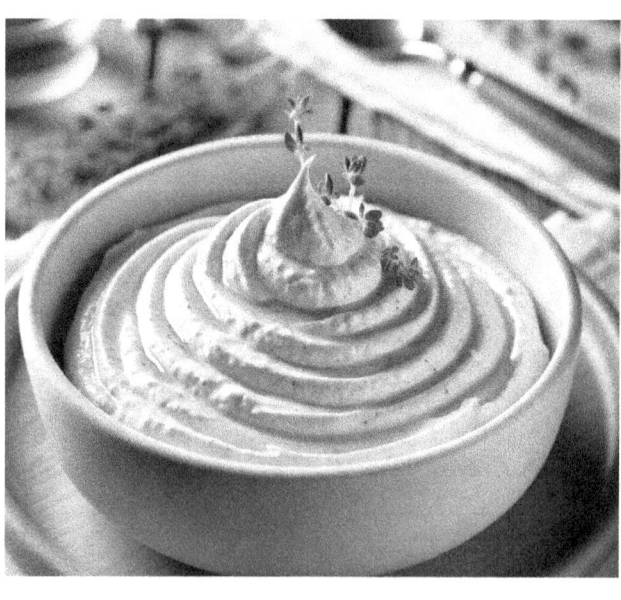

6. Chicken Liver Pate

Ingredients:
- 1 pound chicken livers, trimmed
- 1 small onion, chopped
- 2 garlic cloves, minced
- 1/4 cup low-sodium chicken broth
- 1/4 cup low-fat cream cheese
- 1 teaspoon dried thyme
- 1 tablespoon olive oil

Instructions:
1. Heat the olive oil in a skillet over medium heat.
2. Add the onion and garlic, and sauté until softened, about 5 minutes.
3. Add the chicken livers and cook until no longer pink, about 10 minutes.
4. Transfer the mixture to a blender and add the chicken broth, cream cheese, and thyme.
5. Blend until smooth.
6. Chill in the refrigerator for at least 2 hours before serving.

Nutrition Info (per serving):
- Calories: 150
- Protein: 18g
- Fat: 7g
- Carbohydrates: 3g
- Fiber: 0g
- Sodium: 120mg

Servings: 6 **Cooking Time:** 20 minutes (plus 2 hours chilling time)

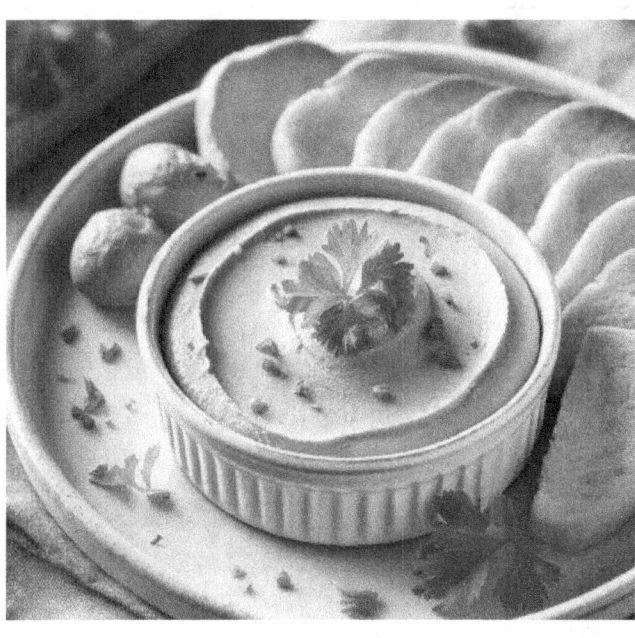

7. Protein-rich Turkey Broth

Ingredients:
- 1 turkey carcass (from a roasted turkey)
- 1 large carrot, chopped
- 1 celery stalk, chopped
- 1 large onion, chopped
- 2 garlic cloves, minced
- 10 cups water
- 1 teaspoon dried thyme
- 1 teaspoon dried rosemary

Instructions:
1. Place the turkey carcass, carrot, celery, onion, and garlic in a large pot.
2. Add the water, thyme, and rosemary.
3. Bring to a boil, then reduce heat and simmer for 3 hours, skimming off any foam.
4. Strain the broth through a fine-mesh sieve.
5. Cool the broth and refrigerate. Skim off any fat that rises to the top.
6. Serve warm.

Nutrition Info (per serving):
- Calories: 60
- Protein: 10g
- Fat: 2g
- Carbohydrates: 2g
- Fiber: 1g
- Sodium: 50mg

Servings: 10 **Cooking Time:** 3 hours

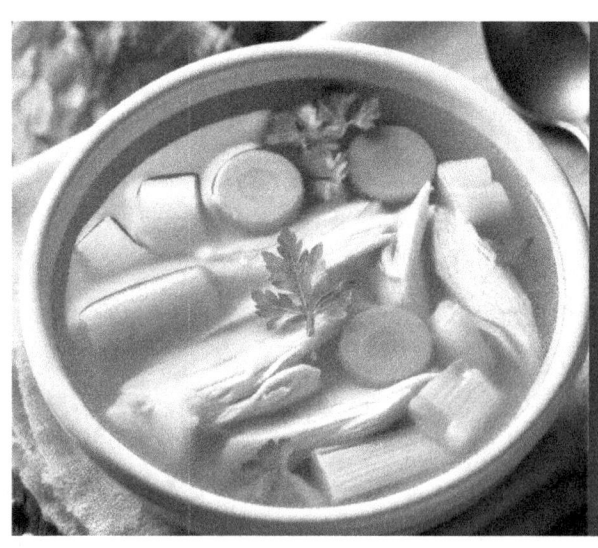

8. Meat Jello

Ingredients:
- 2 cups low-sodium beef broth
- 1 tablespoon unflavored gelatin
- 1/2 cup finely chopped cooked beef
- 1/4 cup finely chopped cooked carrots
- 1/4 cup finely chopped cooked celery

Instructions:
1. In a small bowl, sprinkle the gelatin over 1/2 cup of the beef broth and let it sit for 5 minutes.
2. In a saucepan, heat the remaining 1.5 cups of beef broth until warm.
3. Add the gelatin mixture to the warm broth and stir until completely dissolved.
4. Stir in the chopped beef, carrots, and celery.
5. Pour the mixture into a mold or small dish and refrigerate for at least 2 hours until set.
6. Serve chilled.

Nutrition Info (per serving):
- Calories: 60
- Protein: 10g
- Fat: 2g
- Carbohydrates: 1g
- Fiber: 0g
- Sodium: 150mg

Servings: 4 **Cooking Time:** 2 hours (chilling time)

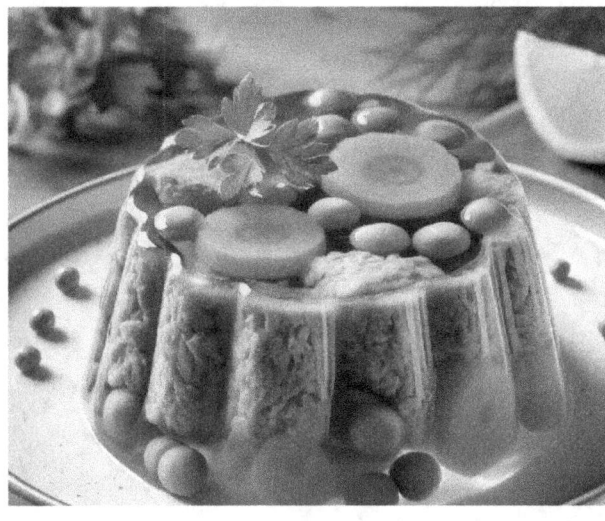

9. Soft Poached Chicken Breast

Ingredients:
- 2 boneless, skinless chicken breasts
- 4 cups low-sodium chicken broth
- 1 bay leaf
- 1 teaspoon dried thyme

Instructions:
1. In a large pot, bring the chicken broth, bay leaf, and thyme to a gentle simmer.
2. Add the chicken breasts to the pot.
3. Poach the chicken for 15-20 minutes until cooked through and tender.
4. Remove the chicken from the broth and let cool slightly before slicing or shredding.
5. Serve warm.

Nutrition Info (per serving):
- Calories: 140
- Protein: 28g
- Fat: 3g
- Carbohydrates: 0g
- Fiber: 0g
- Sodium: 100mg

Servings: 2 **Cooking Time:** 20 minutes

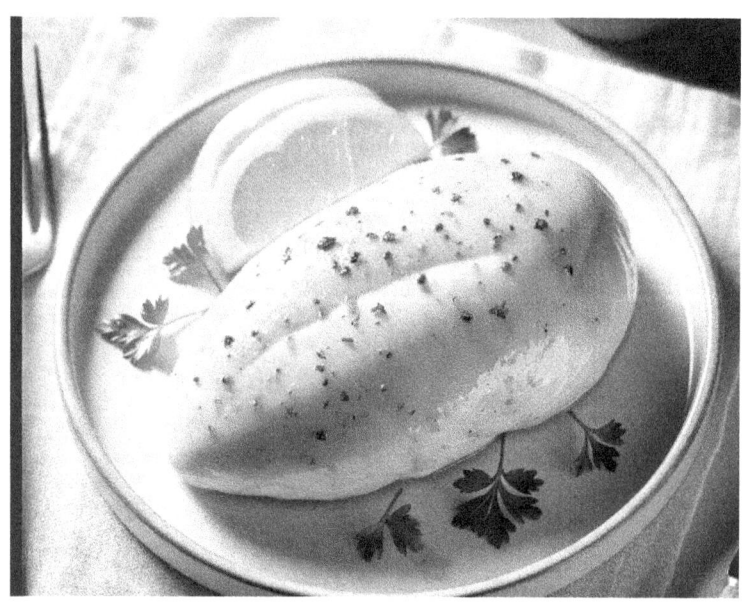

10. Ground Beef Stew

Ingredients:
- 1 pound ground beef
- 1 small onion, chopped
- 2 garlic cloves, minced
- 1 cup chopped carrots
- 1 cup chopped potatoes
- 1 cup chopped celery
- 4 cups low-sodium beef broth
- 1 teaspoon dried thyme
- 1 teaspoon dried oregano

Instructions:
1. In a large pot, cook the ground beef over medium heat until browned.
2. Add the chopped onion and garlic, and sauté until softened, about 5 minutes.
3. Add the carrots, potatoes, celery, beef broth, thyme, and oregano.
4. Bring to a boil, then reduce heat and simmer for 25-30 minutes until the vegetables are tender.
5. Serve warm.

Nutrition Info (per serving):
- Calories: 250
- Protein: 20g
- Fat: 12g
- Carbohydrates: 18g
- Fiber: 3g
- Sodium: 200mg

Servings: 4 **Cooking Time:** 40 minutes

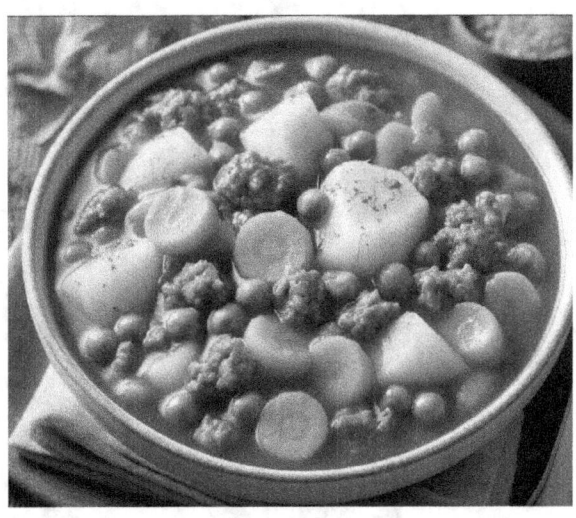

11. Tender Beef Goulash

Ingredients:
- 1 pound beef stew meat, cubed
- 1 small onion, chopped
- 2 garlic cloves, minced
- 1 tablespoon paprika
- 1 teaspoon caraway seeds
- 1 cup low-sodium beef broth
- 1 cup tomato sauce
- 1 bell pepper, chopped

Instructions:
1. In a large pot, cook the beef stew meat over medium heat until browned.
2. Add the chopped onion and garlic, and sauté until softened, about 5 minutes.
3. Stir in the paprika and caraway seeds.
4. Add the beef broth, tomato sauce, and bell pepper.
5. Bring to a boil, then reduce heat and simmer for 1.5 hours until the beef is tender.
6. Serve warm.

Nutrition Info (per serving):
- Calories: 220
- Protein: 25g
- Fat: 10g
- Carbohydrates: 8g
- Fiber: 2g
- Sodium: 250mg

Servings: 4 **Cooking Time:** 1.5 hours

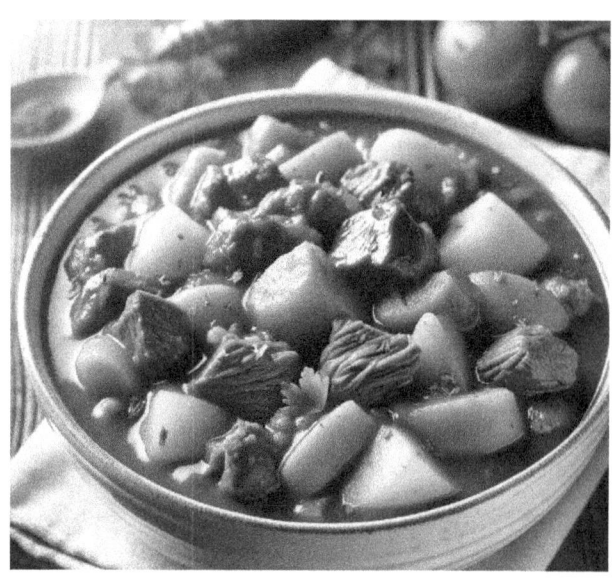

12. Ground Lamb Soup

Ingredients:
- 1 pound ground lamb
- 1 small onion, chopped
- 2 garlic cloves, minced
- 1 cup diced tomatoes (canned, with juice)
- 4 cups low-sodium chicken broth
- 1 cup chopped carrots
- 1 cup chopped zucchini
- 1 teaspoon ground cumin
- 1 teaspoon dried mint

Instructions:
1. In a large pot, cook the ground lamb over medium heat until browned.
2. Add the chopped onion and garlic, and sauté until softened, about 5 minutes.
3. Add the diced tomatoes, chicken broth, carrots, zucchini, cumin, and mint.
4. Bring to a boil, then reduce heat and simmer for 25-30 minutes until the vegetables are tender.
5. Serve warm.

Nutrition Info (per serving):
- Calories: 240
- Protein: 18g
- Fat: 14g
- Carbohydrates: 12g
- Fiber: 3g
- Sodium: 200mg

Servings: 4 **Cooking Time:** 40 minutes

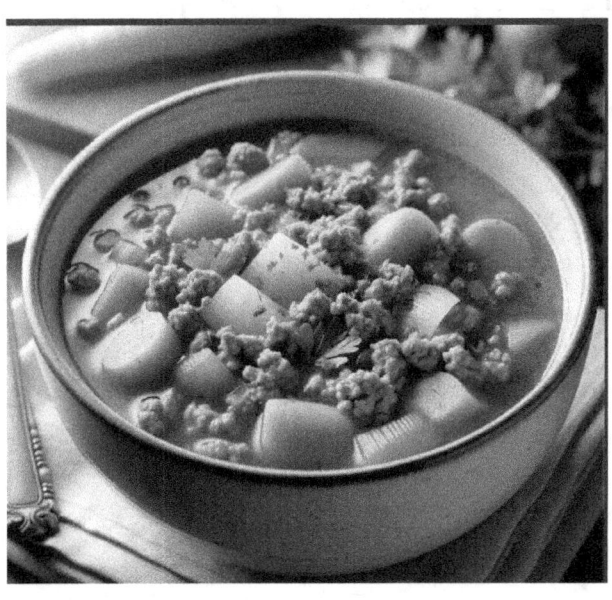

13. Chicken with Mushrooms

Ingredients:
- 4 boneless, skinless chicken breasts
- 1 cup sliced mushrooms
- 1 small onion, chopped
- 1 garlic clove, minced
- 1 cup low-sodium chicken broth
- 1/4 cup low-fat sour cream
- 1 teaspoon dried thyme

Instructions:
1. In a large skillet, cook the chicken breasts over medium heat until browned and cooked through, about 6-7 minutes per side. Remove and set aside.
2. In the same skillet, add the mushrooms, onion, and garlic, and sauté until softened, about 5 minutes.
3. Add the chicken broth and thyme, and bring to a boil.
4. Reduce heat and simmer for 5 minutes.
5. Stir in the sour cream until well combined.
6. Return the chicken to the skillet and heat through.
7. Serve warm.

Nutrition Info (per serving):
- Calories: 180
- Protein: 26g
- Fat: 5g
- Carbohydrates: 4g
- Fiber: 1g
- Sodium: 150mg

Servings: 4 **Cooking Time:** 25 minutes

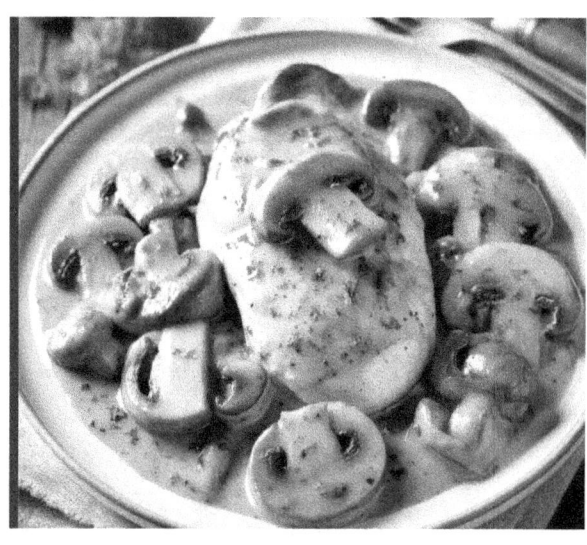

14. Blackened Chicken Breast

Ingredients:
- 4 boneless, skinless chicken breasts
- 1 tablespoon olive oil
- 1 tablespoon paprika
- 1 teaspoon garlic powder
- 1 teaspoon onion powder
- 1/2 teaspoon cayenne pepper

Instructions:
1. Preheat the oven to 375°F (190°C).
2. In a small bowl, mix the paprika, garlic powder, onion powder, and cayenne pepper.
3. Rub the spice mixture over the chicken breasts.
4. Heat the olive oil in an oven-safe skillet over medium-high heat.
5. Cook the chicken breasts for 2-3 minutes per side until blackened.
6. Transfer the skillet to the oven and bake for 15 minutes until the chicken is cooked through.
7. Serve warm.

Nutrition Info (per serving):
- Calories: 180
- Protein: 26g
- Fat: 6g
- Carbohydrates: 1g
- Fiber: 0g
- Sodium: 140mg

Servings: 4 **Cooking Time:** 20 minutes

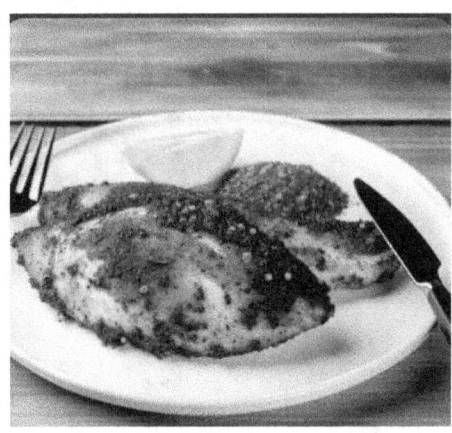

15. Mexicali Meatloaf

Ingredients:
- 1 pound ground beef
- 1/2 cup breadcrumbs
- 1/2 cup salsa
- 1/4 cup chopped green bell pepper
- 1/4 cup chopped onion
- 1 egg, beaten
- 1 teaspoon ground cumin

Instructions:
1. Preheat the oven to 350°F (175°C).
2. In a large bowl, combine the ground beef, breadcrumbs, salsa, green bell pepper, onion, egg, and cumin.
3. Mix until well combined.
4. Shape the mixture into a loaf and place it in a baking dish.
5. Bake for 45-50 minutes until cooked through.
6. Let the meatloaf rest for 10 minutes before slicing.
7. Serve warm.

Nutrition Info (per serving):
- Calories: 220
- Protein: 20g
- Fat: 12g
- Carbohydrates: 8g
- Fiber: 1g
- Sodium: 250mg

Servings: 4 **Cooking Time:** 55 minutes

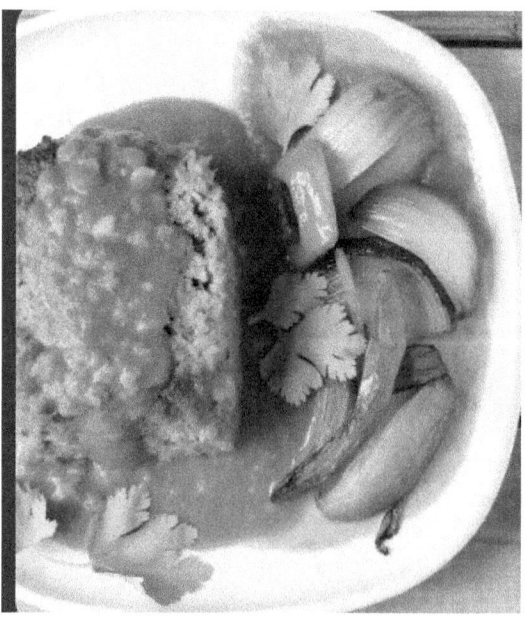

16. Chinese Pork

Ingredients:
- 1 pound pork tenderloin, thinly sliced
- 1/4 cup low-sodium soy sauce
- 2 tablespoons hoisin sauce
- 1 tablespoon rice vinegar
- 1 garlic clove, minced
- 1 teaspoon grated ginger

Instructions:
1. In a bowl, combine the soy sauce, hoisin sauce, rice vinegar, garlic, and ginger.
2. Add the sliced pork and marinate for 30 minutes.
3. Heat a large skillet over medium-high heat.
4. Add the pork and cook for 3-4 minutes per side until cooked through.
5. Serve warm.

Nutrition Info (per serving):
- Calories: 170
- Protein: 25g
- Fat: 5g
- Carbohydrates: 4g
- Fiber: 0g
- Sodium: 300mg

Servings: 4 **Cooking Time:** 40 minutes (including marinating time)

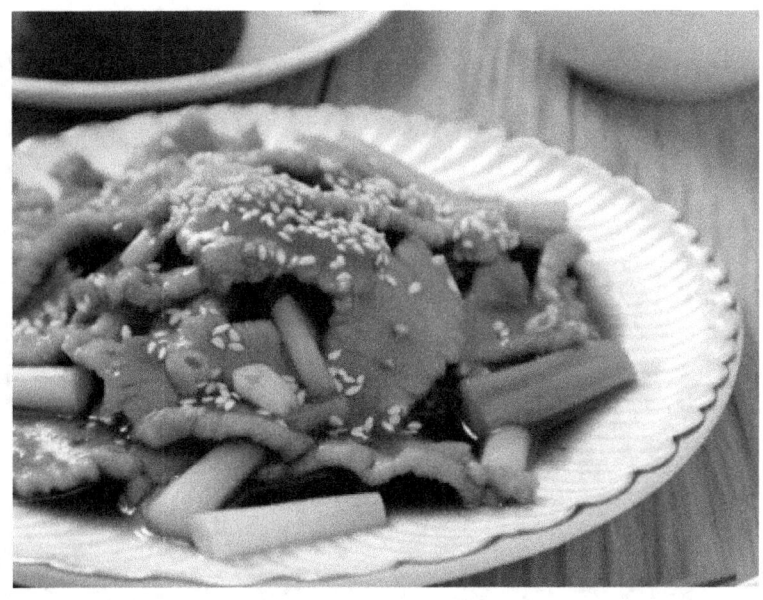

17. Wiener Schnitzel

Ingredients:
- 4 thin slices of veal (or chicken)
- 1/2 cup flour
- 2 eggs, beaten
- 1 cup breadcrumbs
- 2 tablespoons olive oil

Instructions:
1. Place the flour, beaten eggs, and breadcrumbs in separate shallow dishes.
2. Dredge each slice of veal in flour, then dip in the beaten eggs, and finally coat with breadcrumbs.
3. Heat the olive oil in a large skillet over medium-high heat.
4. Cook the veal slices for 2-3 minutes per side until golden brown and cooked through.
5. Serve warm.

Nutrition Info (per serving):
- Calories: 220
- Protein: 18g
- Fat: 10g
- Carbohydrates: 14g
- Fiber: 1g
- Sodium: 200mg

Servings: 4 **Cooking Time:** 10 minutes

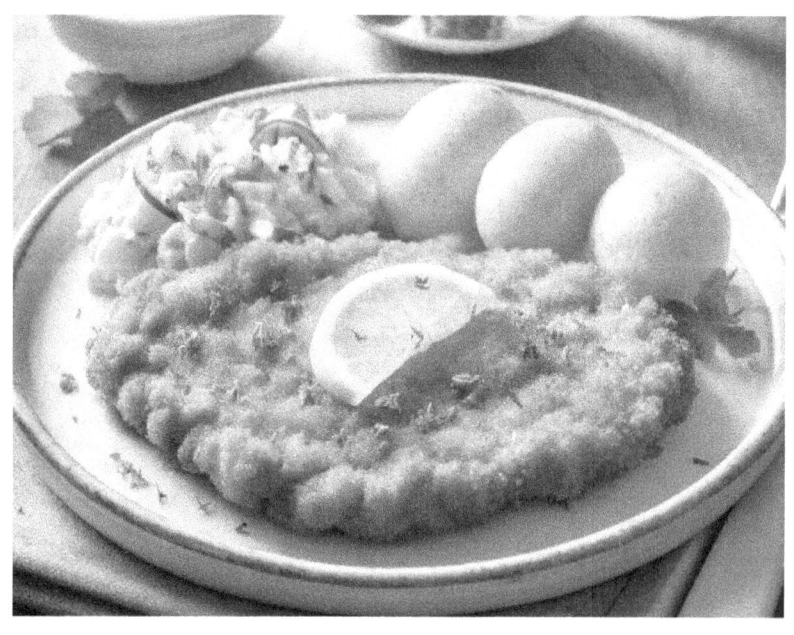

18. Soft Meatballs in Tomato Sauce

Ingredients:
- 1 pound ground beef
- 1/2 cup breadcrumbs
- 1/4 cup grated Parmesan cheese
- 1 egg, beaten
- 1 teaspoon dried oregano
- 2 cups tomato sauce

Instructions:
1. Preheat the oven to 375°F (190°C).
2. In a large bowl, combine the ground beef, breadcrumbs, Parmesan cheese, egg, and oregano.
3. Mix until well combined and shape into small meatballs.
4. Place the meatballs in a baking dish and cover with tomato sauce.
5. Bake for 25-30 minutes until the meatballs are cooked through.
6. Serve warm.

Nutrition Info (per serving):
- Calories: 200
- Protein: 18g
- Fat: 10g
- Carbohydrates: 10g
- Fiber: 2g
- Sodium: 300mg

Servings: 4 **Cooking Time:** 30 minutes

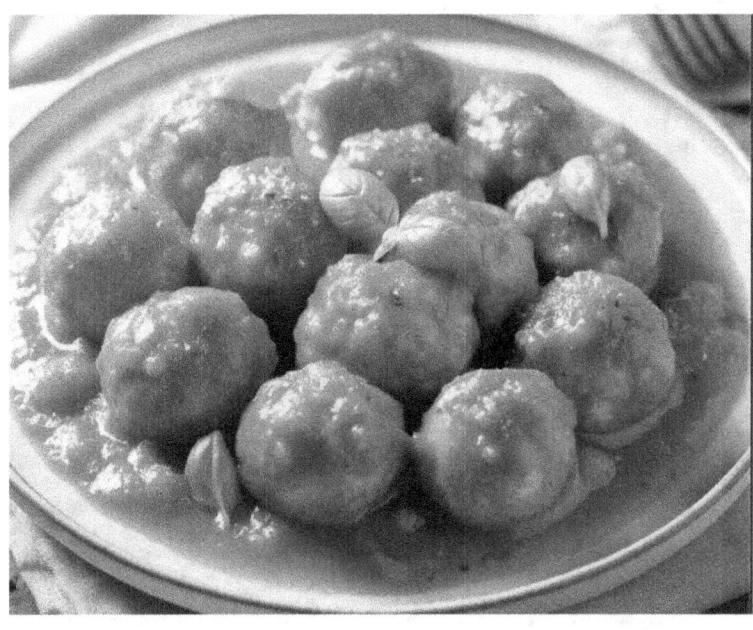

19. Tender Veal Stew

Ingredients:
- 1 pound veal stew meat, cubed
- 1 small onion, chopped
- 2 garlic cloves, minced
- 1 cup chopped carrots
- 1 cup chopped potatoes
- 4 cups low-sodium beef broth
- 1 teaspoon dried thyme
- 1 teaspoon dried rosemary

Instructions:
1. In a large pot, cook the veal stew meat over medium heat until browned.
2. Add the chopped onion and garlic, and sauté until softened, about 5 minutes.
3. Add the carrots, potatoes, beef broth, thyme, and rosemary.
4. Bring to a boil, then reduce heat and simmer for 1.5 hours until the veal is tender.
5. Serve warm.

Nutrition Info (per serving):
- Calories: 220
- Protein: 25g
- Fat: 10g
- Carbohydrates: 12g
- Fiber: 3g
- Sodium: 200mg

Servings: 4 **Cooking Time:** 1.5 hours

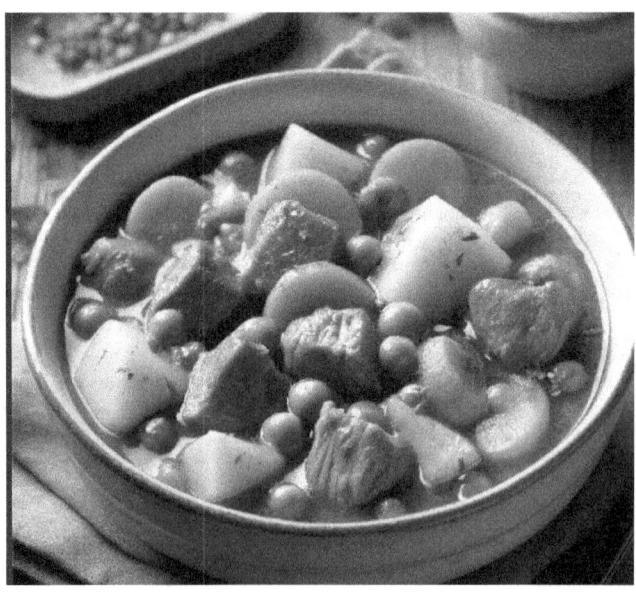

20. Silky Turkey Gravy

Ingredients:
- 2 cups low-sodium turkey broth
- 1/4 cup flour
- 2 tablespoons butter
- 1/2 cup low-fat milk
- 1/2 teaspoon dried sage

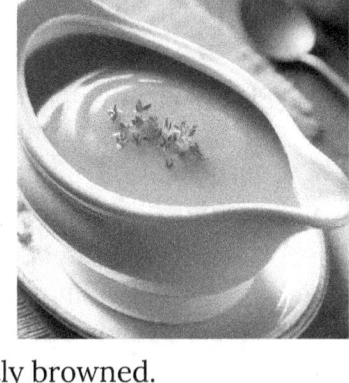

Instructions:
1. In a saucepan, melt the butter over medium heat.
2. Whisk in the flour and cook for 2 minutes until lightly browned.
3. Gradually whisk in the turkey broth and milk.
4. Bring to a simmer and cook for 5-7 minutes until thickened.
5. Stir in the dried sage.
6. Serve warm.

Nutrition Info (per serving):
- Calories: 60
- Protein: 2g
- Fat: 4g
- Carbohydrates: 5g
- Fiber: 0g
- Sodium: 100mg

Servings: 4 **Cooking Time:** 10 minutes

21. Chicken Crepe Filling

Ingredients:
- 1 cup cooked, shredded chicken
- 1/2 cup low-fat ricotta cheese
- 1/4 cup low-fat cream cheese
- 1/4 cup finely chopped spinach
- 1 garlic clove, minced

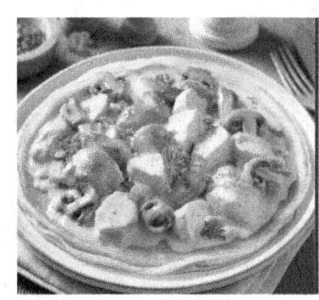

Instructions:
1. In a bowl, combine the shredded chicken, ricotta cheese, cream cheese, spinach, and garlic.
2. Mix until well combined.
3. Use as a filling for crepes.
4. Serve warm.

Nutrition Info (per serving):
- Calories: 100 Protein: 12g Fat: 5g Carbohydrates: 2g Fiber: 0g
- Sodium: 120mg

Servings: 4 **Cooking Time:** 5 minutes

22. Mild Meat Chili

Ingredients:
- 1 pound ground beef
- 1 small onion, chopped
- 2 garlic cloves, minced
- 1 cup diced tomatoes (canned, with juice)
- 1 cup low-sodium beef broth
- 1 cup cooked kidney beans
- 1 tablespoon chili powder
- 1 teaspoon ground cumin

Instructions:
1. In a large pot, cook the ground beef over medium heat until browned.
2. Add the chopped onion and garlic, and sauté until softened, about 5 minutes.
3. Add the diced tomatoes, beef broth, kidney beans, chili powder, and cumin.
4. Bring to a boil, then reduce heat and simmer for 25-30 minutes.
5. Serve warm.

Nutrition Info (per serving):
- Calories: 240
- Protein: 20g
- Fat: 12g
- Carbohydrates: 12g
- Fiber: 4g
- Sodium: 200mg

Servings: 4 **Cooking Time:** 40 minutes

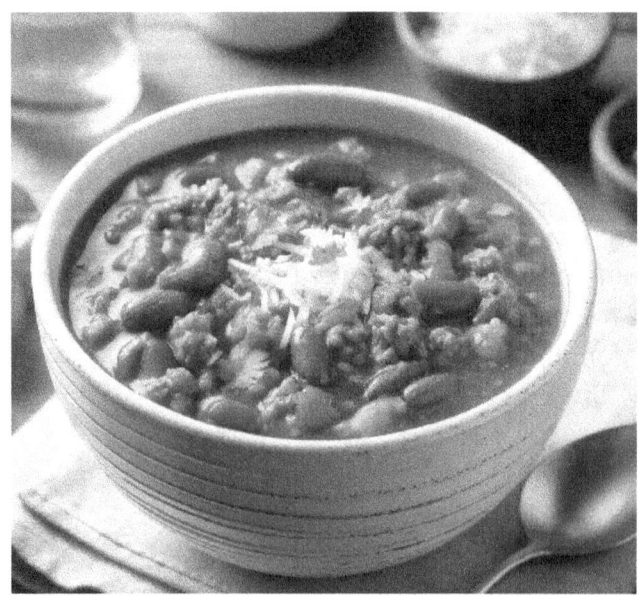

23. Pureed Liver with Onion

Ingredients:
- 1 pound chicken livers, trimmed
- 1 small onion, chopped
- 2 garlic cloves, minced
- 1/4 cup low-sodium chicken broth
- 1/4 cup low-fat cream cheese
- 1 tablespoon olive oil

Instructions:
1. Heat the olive oil in a skillet over medium heat.
2. Add the onion and garlic, and sauté until softened, about 5 minutes.
3. Add the chicken livers and cook until no longer pink, about 10 minutes.
4. Transfer the mixture to a blender and add the chicken broth and cream cheese.
5. Blend until smooth.
6. Serve warm.

Nutrition Info (per serving):
- Calories: 150
- Protein: 18g
- Fat: 7g
- Carbohydrates: 3g
- Fiber: 0g
- Sodium: 120mg

Servings: 6 **Cooking Time:** 20 minutes

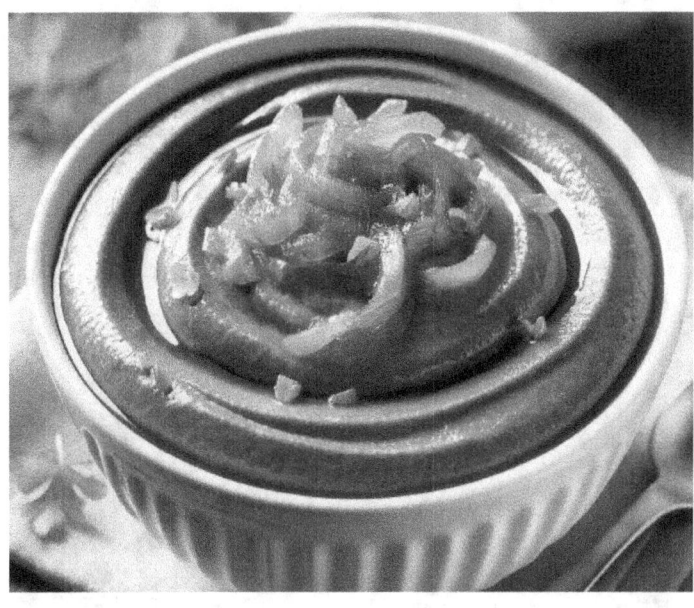

24. Tender Stewed Rabbit

Ingredients:
- 1 rabbit, cut into pieces
- 1 small onion, chopped
- 2 garlic cloves, minced
- 1 cup chopped carrots
- 1 cup chopped potatoes
- 4 cups low-sodium chicken broth
- 1 teaspoon dried thyme
- 1 teaspoon dried rosemary

Instructions:
1. In a large pot, cook the rabbit pieces over medium heat until browned.
2. Add the chopped onion and garlic, and sauté until softened, about 5 minutes.
3. Add the carrots, potatoes, chicken broth, thyme, and rosemary.
4. Bring to a boil, then reduce heat and simmer for 1.5 hours until the rabbit is tender.
5. Serve warm.

Nutrition Info (per serving):
- Calories: 220
- Protein: 25g
- Fat: 10g
- Carbohydrates: 12g
- Fiber: 3g
- Sodium: 200mg

Servings: 4 **Cooking Time:** 1.5 hours

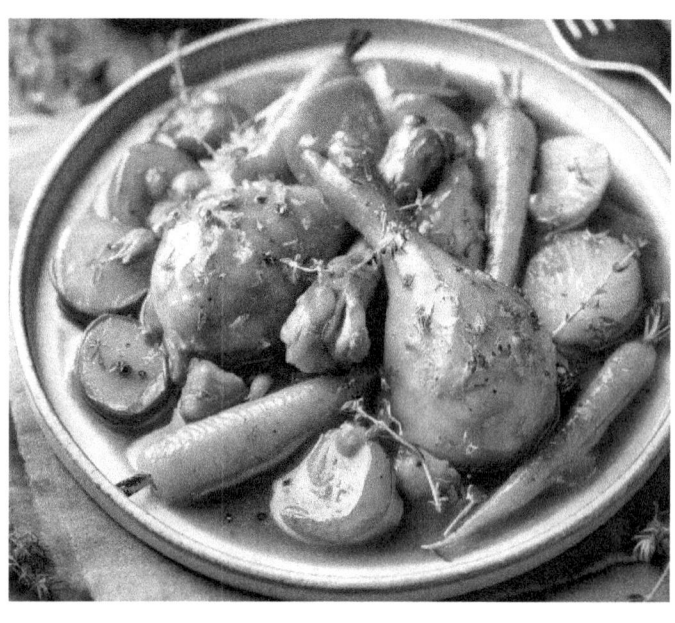

25. Chicken and Yogurt Soup

Ingredients:
- 2 cups cooked, shredded chicken
- 4 cups low-sodium chicken broth
- 1 cup plain low-fat yogurt
- 1/2 cup finely chopped carrots
- 1/2 cup finely chopped celery
- 1/2 teaspoon ground turmeric

Instructions:
1. In a large pot, bring the chicken broth to a boil.
2. Add the shredded chicken, chopped carrots, and chopped celery.
3. Reduce heat and simmer for 15 minutes until the vegetables are tender.
4. Stir in the yogurt and turmeric.
5. Cook for an additional 5 minutes.
6. Serve warm.

Nutrition Info (per serving):
- Calories: 150
- Protein: 20g
- Fat: 4g
- Carbohydrates: 8g
- Fiber: 1g
- Sodium: 150mg

Servings: 4 **Cooking Time:** 25 minutes

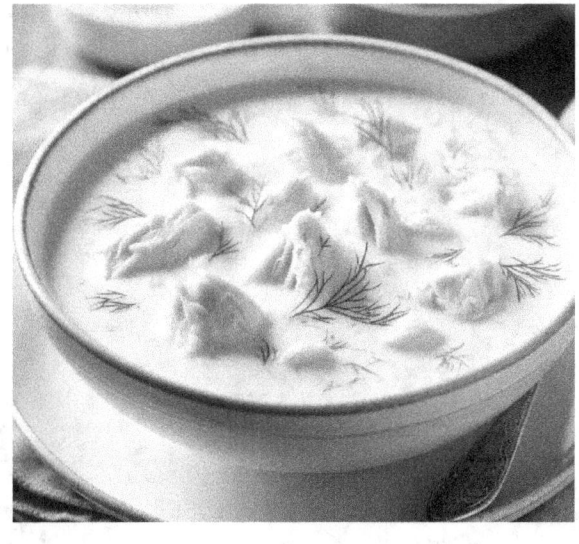

Fish and Seafood Recipes

1. Pureed White Fish
Ingredients:
- 1 pound white fish fillets (such as cod or haddock), cooked and flaked
- 1 cup low-sodium fish or vegetable broth
- 1/4 cup low-fat cream cheese
- 1 tablespoon lemon juice

Instructions:
1. Place the cooked and flaked fish in a blender or food processor.
2. Add the broth, cream cheese, and lemon juice.
3. Blend until smooth.
4. Serve warm or chilled.

Nutrition Info (per serving):
- Calories: 150
- Protein: 26g
- Fat: 4g
- Carbohydrates: 2g
- Fiber: 0g
- Sodium: 150mg

Servings: 4 **Cooking Time:** 10 minutes

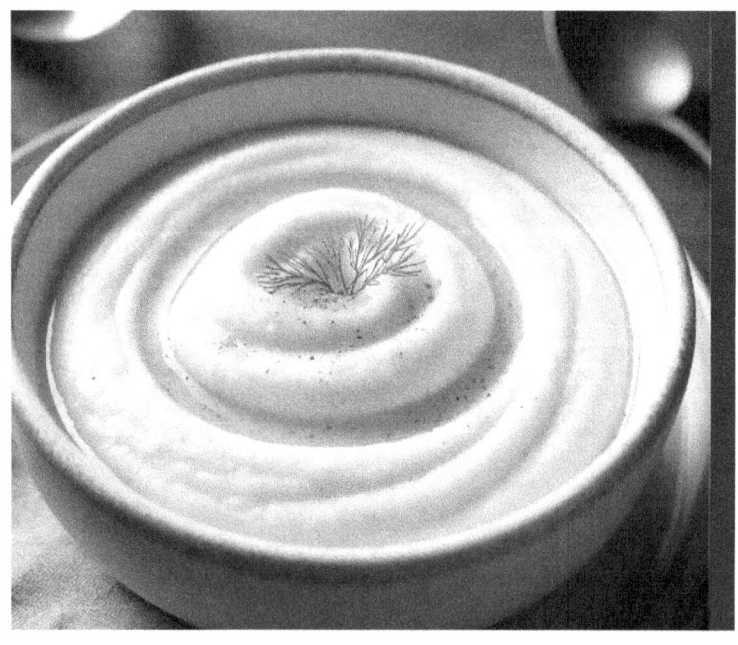

2. Soft Salmon Mousse

Ingredients:
- 1 pound cooked salmon, flaked
- 1/2 cup low-fat Greek yogurt
- 1 tablespoon lemon juice
- 1 teaspoon Dijon mustard

Instructions:
1. Place the flaked salmon in a blender or food processor.
2. Add the Greek yogurt, lemon juice, and Dijon mustard.
3. Blend until smooth.
4. Serve chilled.

Nutrition Info (per serving):
- Calories: 180
- Protein: 25g
- Fat: 7g
- Carbohydrates: 2g
- Fiber: 0g
- Sodium: 100mg

Servings: 4 **Cooking Time:** 10 minutes

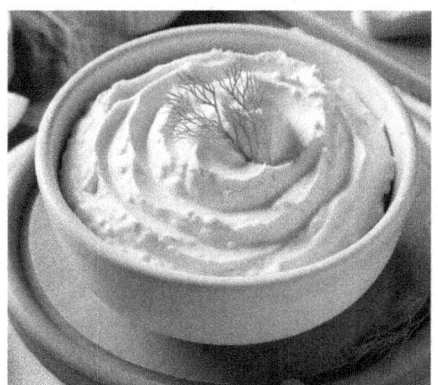

3. Tender Flaked Tuna

Ingredients:
- 2 cans (5 ounces each) tuna packed in water, drained
- 1/4 cup low-fat mayonnaise
- 1 tablespoon lemon juice
- 1 teaspoon Dijon mustard

Instructions:
1. Place the drained tuna in a bowl.
2. Add the mayonnaise, lemon juice, and Dijon mustard.
3. Mix until well combined and the tuna is flaked.
4. Serve chilled.

Nutrition Info (per serving):
- Calories: 150
- Protein: 22g
- Fat: 5g
- Carbohydrates: 1g
- Fiber: 0g
- Sodium: 200mg

Servings: 4 **Cooking Time:** 5 minutes

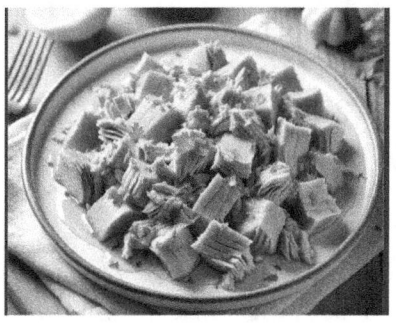

4. Paprika Shrimp Puree

Ingredients:
- 1 pound cooked shrimp, peeled and deveined
- 1/2 cup low-sodium chicken broth
- 1/4 cup low-fat cream cheese
- 1 teaspoon paprika

Instructions:
1. Place the cooked shrimp in a blender or food processor.
2. Add the chicken broth, cream cheese, and paprika.
3. Blend until smooth.
4. Serve warm or chilled.

Nutrition Info (per serving):
- Calories: 150
- Protein: 22g
- Fat: 4g
- Carbohydrates: 2g
- Fiber: 0g
- Sodium: 200mg

Servings: 4 **Cooking Time:** 10 minutes

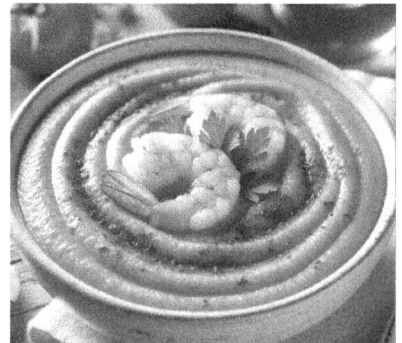

5. Silky Lobster Bisque

Ingredients:
- 1 pound cooked lobster meat, chopped
- 2 cups low-sodium fish or vegetable broth
- 1/2 cup low-fat milk
- 1/4 cup low-fat cream cheese
- 1 tablespoon tomato paste

Instructions:
1. In a pot, heat the fish or vegetable broth over medium heat.
2. Add the chopped lobster meat, milk, cream cheese, and tomato paste.
3. Simmer for 10 minutes, stirring occasionally.
4. Use an immersion blender to blend until smooth.
5. Serve warm.

Nutrition Info (per serving):
- Calories: 200
- Protein: 25g
- Fat: 7g
- Carbohydrates: 4g
- Fiber: 0g
- Sodium: 300mg

Servings: 4 **Cooking Time:** 20 minutes

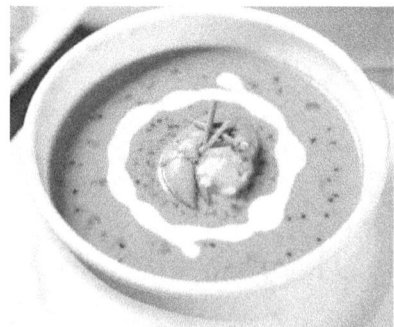

6. Sole in White Sauce

Ingredients:
- 1 pound sole fillets, cooked and flaked
- 1 cup low-fat milk
- 1/4 cup low-fat cream cheese
- 1 tablespoon lemon juice
- 1/2 teaspoon garlic powder

Instructions:
1. In a pot, heat the milk over medium heat.
2. Add the flaked sole, cream cheese, lemon juice, and garlic powder.
3. Simmer for 5 minutes, stirring occasionally.
4. Use an immersion blender to blend until smooth.
5. Serve warm.

Nutrition Info (per serving):
- Calories: 160
- Protein: 28g
- Fat: 4g
- Carbohydrates: 2g
- Fiber: 0g
- Sodium: 200mg

Servings: 4 **Cooking Time:** 10 minutes

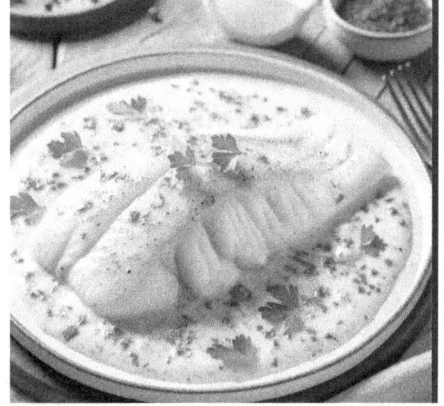

7. Scallop Pate

Ingredients:
- 1 pound cooked scallops
- 1/4 cup low-fat cream cheese
- 1 tablespoon lemon juice
- 1 teaspoon Dijon mustard

Instructions:
1. Place the cooked scallops in a blender or food processor.
2. Add the cream cheese, lemon juice, and Dijon mustard.
3. Blend until smooth.
4. Serve chilled.

Nutrition Info (per serving):
- Calories: 160
- Protein: 24g
- Fat: 4g
- Carbohydrates: 3g
- Fiber: 0g
- Sodium: 250mg

Servings: 4 **Cooking Time:** 10 minutes

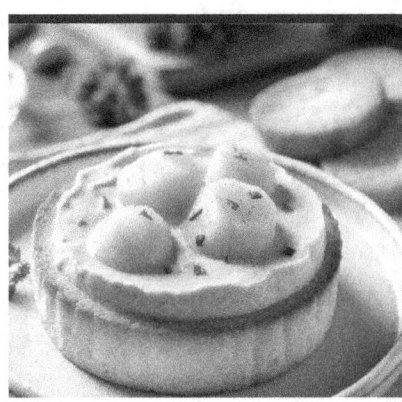

8. Mashed Anchovies

Ingredients:
- 1 can (2 ounces) anchovies, drained
- 1/4 cup low-fat cream cheese
- 1 tablespoon lemon juice
- 1 teaspoon chopped fresh parsley

Instructions:
1. Place the drained anchovies in a bowl.
2. Add the cream cheese, lemon juice, and chopped parsley.
3. Mash with a fork until smooth.
4. Serve chilled.

Nutrition Info (per serving):
- Calories: 100
- Protein: 6g
- Fat: 7g
- Carbohydrates: 1g
- Fiber: 0g
- Sodium: 400mg

Servings: 4 **Cooking Time:** 5 minutes

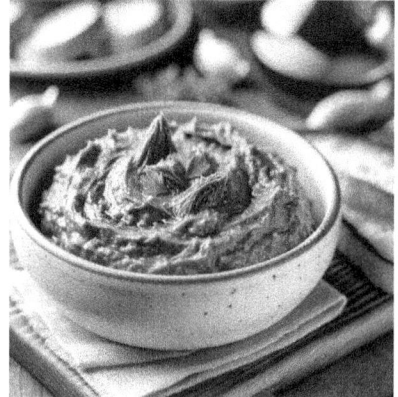

9. Tilapia Puree

Ingredients:
- 1 pound tilapia fillets, cooked and flaked
- 1 cup low-sodium vegetable broth
- 1/4 cup low-fat Greek yogurt
- 1 tablespoon lemon juice

Instructions:
1. Place the cooked and flaked tilapia in a blender or food processor.
2. Add the vegetable broth, Greek yogurt, and lemon juice.
3. Blend until smooth.
4. Serve warm or chilled.

Nutrition Info (per serving):
- Calories: 140
- Protein: 26g
- Fat: 3g
- Carbohydrates: 2g
- Fiber: 0g
- Sodium: 150mg

Servings: 4 **Cooking Time:** 10 minutes

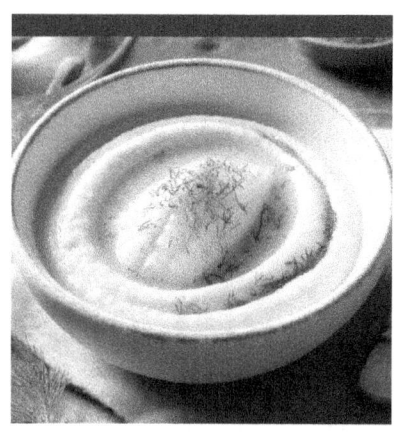

10. Creamy Salmon Spread

Ingredients:
- 1 pound cooked salmon, flaked
- 1/4 cup low-fat cream cheese
- 2 tablespoons low-fat Greek yogurt
- 1 tablespoon lemon juice
- 1 teaspoon dill

Instructions:
1. Place the flaked salmon in a bowl.
2. Add the cream cheese, Greek yogurt, lemon juice, and dill.
3. Mix until well combined and smooth.
4. Serve chilled.

Nutrition Info (per serving):
- Calories: 160
- Protein: 24g
- Fat: 6g
- Carbohydrates: 2g
- Fiber: 0g
- Sodium: 100mg

Servings: 4 **Cooking Time:** 10 minutes

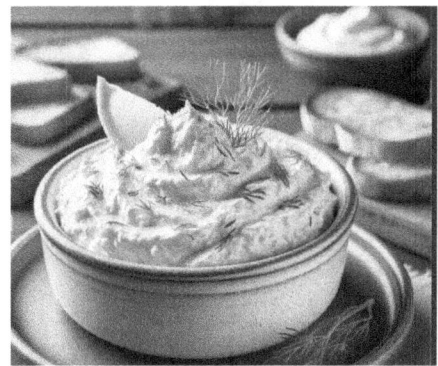

11. Flounder and Parsley Soup

Ingredients:
- 1 pound flounder fillets, cooked and flaked
- 4 cups low-sodium fish or vegetable broth
- 1/2 cup chopped fresh parsley
- 1/2 cup low-fat milk

Instructions:
1. In a pot, heat the fish or vegetable broth over medium heat.
2. Add the flaked flounder, chopped parsley, and milk.
3. Simmer for 10 minutes, stirring occasionally.
4. Use an immersion blender to blend until smooth.
5. Serve warm.

Nutrition Info (per serving):
- Calories: 140
- Protein: 24g
- Fat: 3g
- Carbohydrates: 2g
- Fiber: 1g
- Sodium: 150mg

Servings: 4 **Cooking Time:** 15 minutes

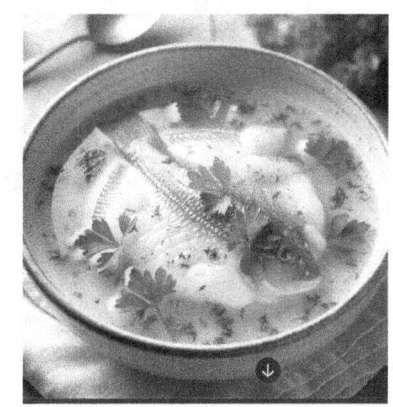

12. Shrimp and Cucumber Gel

Ingredients:
- 1 pound cooked shrimp, peeled and deveined
- 1 cup peeled and diced cucumber
- 1 cup low-sodium vegetable broth
- 1 tablespoon unflavored gelatin
- 1 tablespoon lemon juice

Instructions:
1. In a small bowl, sprinkle the gelatin over 1/2 cup of the vegetable broth and let it sit for 5 minutes.
2. In a saucepan, heat the remaining 1/2 cup of vegetable broth until warm.
3. Add the gelatin mixture to the warm broth and stir until completely dissolved.
4. Place the cooked shrimp and diced cucumber in a blender or food processor.
5. Add the lemon juice and the gelatin mixture.
6. Blend until smooth.
7. Pour the mixture into a mold or small dish and refrigerate for at least 2 hours until set.
8. Serve chilled.

Nutrition Info (per serving):
- Calories: 150
- Protein: 24g
- Fat: 2g
- Carbohydrates: 3g
- Fiber: 0g
- Sodium: 200mg

Servings: 4 **Cooking Time:** 2 hours (chilling time)

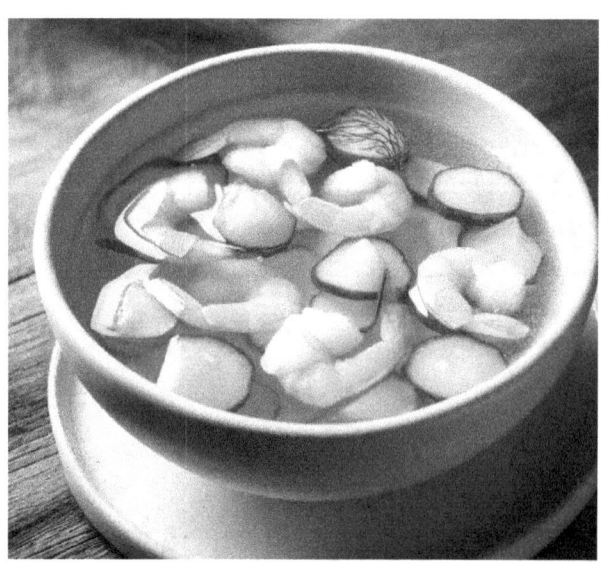

14. Mild Mackerel Puree

Ingredients:
- 1 pound cooked mackerel fillets, flaked
- 1 cup low-sodium fish broth
- 1/4 cup low-fat Greek yogurt
- 1 tablespoon lemon juice

Instructions:
1. Place the cooked and flaked mackerel in a blender or food processor.
2. Add the fish broth, Greek yogurt, and lemon juice.
3. Blend until smooth.
4. Serve warm or chilled.

Nutrition Info (per serving):
- Calories: 180
- Protein: 28g
- Fat: 6g
- Carbohydrates: 2g
- Fiber: 0g
- Sodium: 200mg

Servings: 4 **Cooking Time:** 10 minutes

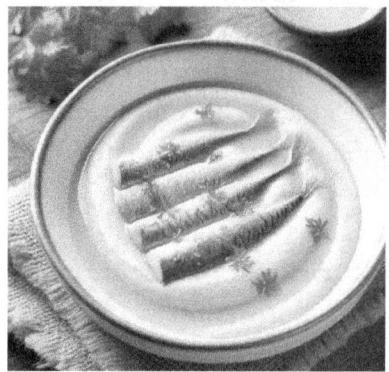

15. Tuna and Sweet Potato Mash

Ingredients:
- 1 can (5 ounces) tuna packed in water, drained
- 1 large sweet potato, peeled and cubed
- 1/4 cup low-fat milk
- 1 tablespoon olive oil

Instructions:
1. Boil the sweet potato in a pot of water until tender, about 15 minutes.
2. Drain the sweet potato and place it in a bowl.
3. Add the drained tuna, milk, and olive oil.
4. Mash until smooth and well combined.
5. Serve warm.

Nutrition Info (per serving):
- Calories: 200
- Protein: 18g
- Fat: 6g
- Carbohydrates: 22g
- Fiber: 4g
- Sodium: 250mg

Servings: 2 **Cooking Time:** 20 minutes

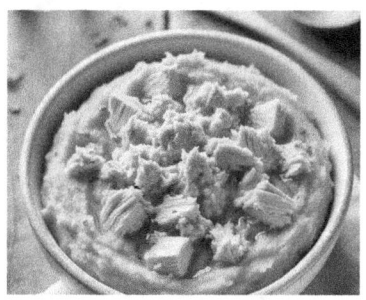

16. Catfish Soup

Ingredients:
- 1 pound catfish fillets, cubed
- 1 small onion, chopped
- 1 garlic clove, minced
- 1 cup chopped celery
- 1 cup chopped carrots
- 4 cups low-sodium chicken broth
- 1 teaspoon dried thyme

Instructions:
1. In a large pot, sauté the onion and garlic until softened, about 5 minutes.
2. Add the celery and carrots, and sauté for another 5 minutes.
3. Add the chicken broth and thyme, and bring to a boil.
4. Reduce heat and simmer for 10 minutes.
5. Add the cubed catfish and cook for an additional 5-7 minutes until the fish is cooked through.
6. Serve warm.

Nutrition Info (per serving):
- Calories: 160
- Protein: 24g
- Fat: 4g
- Carbohydrates: 8g
- Fiber: 2g
- Sodium: 150mg

Servings: 4 **Cooking Time:** 25 minutes

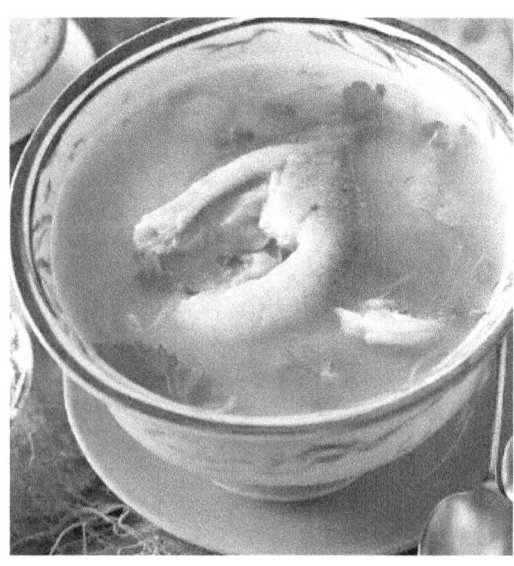

17. Haddock in Mustard Sauce

Ingredients:
- 1 pound haddock fillets, cooked and flaked
- 1/2 cup low-fat Greek yogurt
- 2 tablespoons Dijon mustard
- 1 tablespoon lemon juice

Instructions:
1. Place the cooked and flaked haddock in a bowl.
2. In a separate bowl, mix the Greek yogurt, Dijon mustard, and lemon juice.
3. Pour the mustard sauce over the haddock and mix until well combined.
4. Serve warm or chilled.

Nutrition Info (per serving):
- Calories: 170
- Protein: 28g
- Fat: 4g
- Carbohydrates: 3g
- Fiber: 0g
- Sodium: 250mg

Servings: 4 **Cooking Time:** 10 minutes

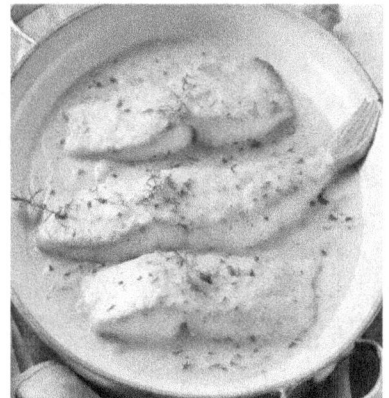

18. Barramundi Broth

Ingredients:
- 1 pound barramundi fillets, cooked and flaked
- 4 cups low-sodium fish broth
- 1/2 cup chopped celery
- 1/2 cup chopped leeks
- 1 tablespoon lemon juice
- 1 teaspoon dried dill

Instructions:
1. In a large pot, heat the fish broth over medium heat.
2. Add the chopped celery and leeks, and simmer for 10 minutes until tender.
3. Add the flaked barramundi, lemon juice, and dried dill.
4. Cook for an additional 5 minutes.
5. Serve warm.

Nutrition Info (per serving):
- Calories: 140
- Protein: 25g
- Fat: 3g
- Carbohydrates: 2g
- Fiber: 1g
- Sodium: 150mg

Servings: 4 **Cooking Time:** 20 minutes

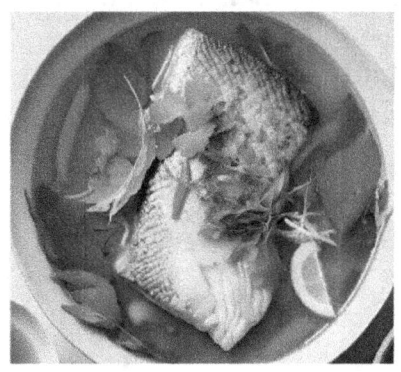

19. Snapper and Carrot Soup

Ingredients:
- 1 pound snapper fillets, cooked and flaked
- 1 cup chopped carrots
- 1 small onion, chopped
- 2 garlic cloves, minced
- 4 cups low-sodium vegetable broth
- 1 teaspoon dried basil

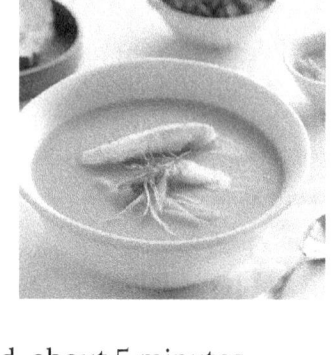

Instructions:
1. In a large pot, sauté the onion and garlic until softened, about 5 minutes.
2. Add the chopped carrots and sauté for another 5 minutes.
3. Add the vegetable broth and dried basil, and bring to a boil.
4. Reduce heat and simmer for 10 minutes.
5. Add the flaked snapper and cook for an additional 5 minutes.
6. Serve warm.

Nutrition Info (per serving):
- Calories: 150 Protein: 24g Fat: 3g Carbohydrates: 6g
- Fiber: 2g
- Sodium: 150mg

Servings: 4 **Cooking Time:** 25 minutes

20. Mullet in Light Broth

Ingredients:
- 1 pound mullet fillets, cooked and flaked
- 4 cups low-sodium fish broth
- 1/2 cup chopped celery
- 1/2 cup chopped fennel
- 1 tablespoon lemon juice
- 1 teaspoon dried thyme

Instructions:
1. In a large pot, heat the fish broth over medium heat.
2. Add the chopped celery and fennel, and simmer for 10 minutes until tender.
3. Add the flaked mullet, lemon juice, and dried thyme.
4. Cook for an additional 5 minutes.
5. Serve warm.

Nutrition Info (per serving):
- Calories: 140
- Protein: 24g
- Fat: 3g
- Carbohydrates: 2g
- Fiber: 1g
- Sodium: 150mg

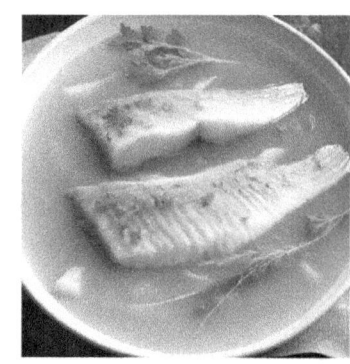

Servings: 4 **Cooking Time:** 20 minutes

21. Crawfish Tail Mix

Ingredients:
- 1 pound cooked crawfish tails
- 1/2 cup low-fat Greek yogurt
- 1 tablespoon lemon juice
- 1 teaspoon Dijon mustard
- 1/4 cup finely chopped green onions

Instructions:
1. Place the cooked crawfish tails in a bowl.
2. In a separate bowl, mix the Greek yogurt, lemon juice, Dijon mustard, and chopped green onions.
3. Pour the yogurt mixture over the crawfish tails and mix until well combined.
4. Serve chilled.

Nutrition Info (per serving):
- Calories: 150
- Protein: 24g
- Fat: 4g
- Carbohydrates: 2g
- Fiber: 0g
- Sodium: 200mg

Servings: 4 **Cooking Time:** 10 minutes

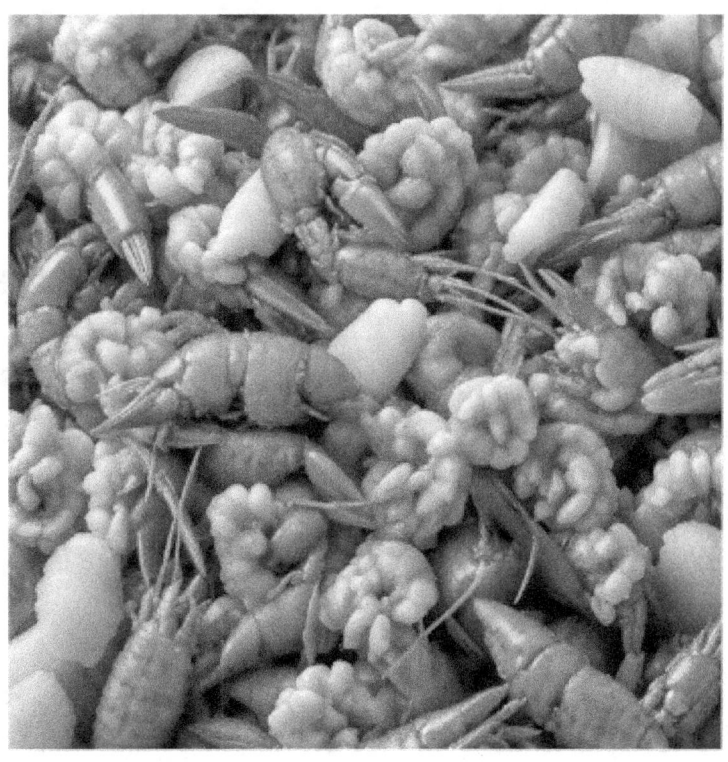

Soup & Stew Recipes

1. Chicken and Thyme Broth
Ingredients:
- 1 whole chicken (about 3-4 pounds)
- 2 large carrots, peeled and chopped
- 2 celery stalks, chopped
- 1 large onion, chopped
- 2 garlic cloves, minced
- 1 bay leaf
- 1 teaspoon dried thyme
- 10 cups water

Instructions:
1. Place the chicken in a large pot.
2. Add the carrots, celery, onion, garlic, bay leaf, and thyme.
3. Pour in the water and bring to a boil over high heat.
4. Reduce the heat to low and simmer for 3 hours, skimming off any foam that rises to the top.
5. Remove the chicken and vegetables from the broth. Discard the vegetables.
6. Strain the broth through a fine-mesh sieve into another pot or large bowl.
7. Serve warm.

Nutrition Info (per serving):
- Calories: 80
- Protein: 10g
- Fat: 3g
- Carbohydrates: 1g
- Fiber: 0g
- Sodium: 150mg

Servings: 10 **Cooking Time:** 3 hours 15 minutes

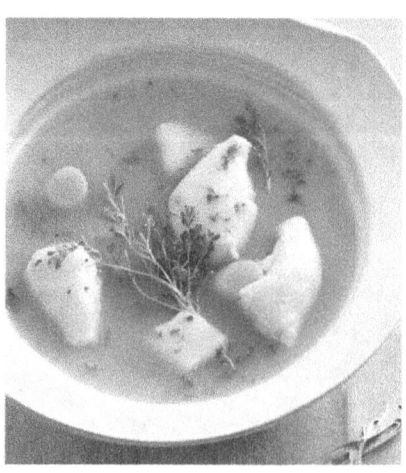

2. Turkey and Sage Soup

Ingredients:
- 1 pound ground turkey
- 1 small onion, chopped
- 2 garlic cloves, minced
- 2 cups chopped carrots
- 2 cups chopped celery
- 4 cups low-sodium chicken broth
- 1 teaspoon dried sage
- 1 cup cooked wild rice

Instructions:
1. In a large pot, cook the ground turkey over medium heat until browned.
2. Add the chopped onion and garlic, and sauté until softened, about 5 minutes.
3. Add the carrots, celery, chicken broth, and sage.
4. Bring to a boil, then reduce heat and simmer for 20 minutes.
5. Stir in the cooked wild rice and cook for an additional 5 minutes.
6. Serve warm.

Nutrition Info (per serving):
- Calories: 200 Protein: 20g Fat: 6g Carbohydrates: 18g
- Fiber: 3g
- Sodium: 150mg

Servings: 6 **Cooking Time:** 35 minutes

3. Lentil and Ham Soup

Ingredients:
- 1 cup dried lentils, rinsed
- 1 cup diced ham
- 1 small onion, chopped
- 2 garlic cloves, minced
- 2 cups chopped carrots
- 2 cups chopped celery
- 4 cups low-sodium chicken broth
- 1 teaspoon dried thyme

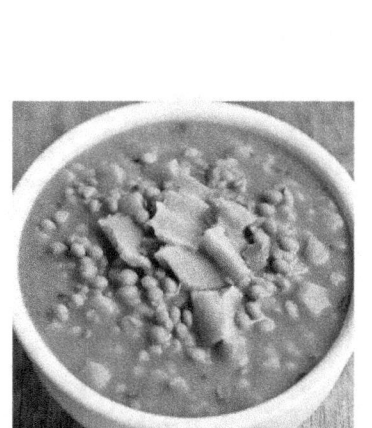

Instructions:
1. In a large pot, sauté the onion and garlic until softened, about 5 minutes.
2. Add the carrots, celery, lentils, ham, chicken broth, and thyme.
3. Bring to a boil, then reduce heat and simmer for 30 minutes until the lentils are tender.
4. Serve warm.

Nutrition Info (per serving):
Calories: 220 Protein: 18g Fat: 4g Carbohydrates: 28g Fiber: 10g Sodium: 200mg
Servings: 6 **Cooking Time:** 40 minutes

4. Pea and Mint Soup

Ingredients:
- 4 cups frozen peas
- 1 small onion, chopped
- 2 garlic cloves, minced
- 4 cups low-sodium vegetable broth
- 1/4 cup fresh mint leaves
- 1/2 cup low-fat Greek yogurt

Instructions:
1. In a large pot, sauté the onion and garlic until softened, about 5 minutes.
2. Add the peas and vegetable broth, and bring to a boil.
3. Reduce heat and simmer for 10 minutes.
4. Stir in the mint leaves.
5. Use an immersion blender to blend the soup until smooth.
6. Stir in the Greek yogurt.
7. Serve warm.

Nutrition Info (per serving):
- Calories: 150
- Protein: 10g
- Fat: 2g
- Carbohydrates: 25g
- Fiber: 8g
- Sodium: 200mg

Servings: 4 **Cooking Time:** 20 minutes

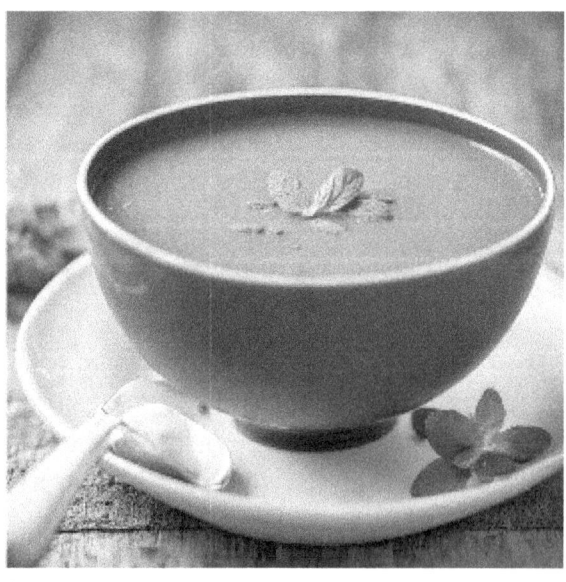

5. Silky Egg Drop Soup

Ingredients:
- 4 cups low-sodium chicken broth
- 2 large eggs, beaten
- 1 tablespoon cornstarch
- 1 tablespoon water
- 1 teaspoon grated ginger
- 1/4 cup chopped green onions

Instructions:
1. In a large pot, bring the chicken broth to a boil.
2. Mix the cornstarch and water to create a slurry, and stir it into the boiling broth.
3. Reduce heat to a simmer and add the grated ginger.
4. Slowly pour the beaten eggs into the broth while stirring continuously to create egg ribbons.
5. Simmer for 2 minutes until the eggs are cooked.
6. Garnish with chopped green onions.
7. Serve warm.

Nutrition Info (per serving):
- Calories: 80
- Protein: 8g
- Fat: 3g
- Carbohydrates: 5g
- Fiber: 0g
- Sodium: 150mg

Servings: 4 **Cooking Time:** 10 minutes

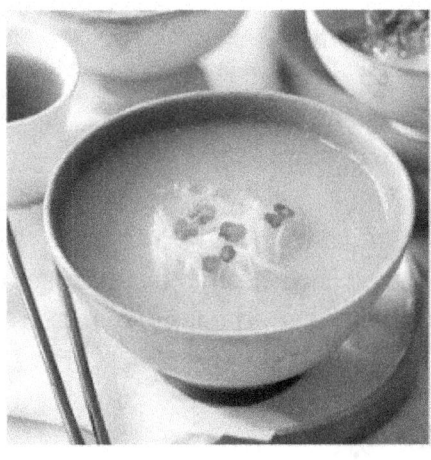

6. Quinoa and Vegetable Stew

Ingredients:
- 1 cup quinoa, rinsed
- 1 small onion, chopped
- 2 garlic cloves, minced
- 2 cups chopped carrots
- 2 cups chopped zucchini
- 4 cups low-sodium vegetable broth
- 1 teaspoon dried oregano
- 1 teaspoon dried basil
- 1/2 cup chopped spinach

Instructions:
1. In a large pot, sauté the onion and garlic until softened, about 5 minutes.
2. Add the carrots, zucchini, quinoa, vegetable broth, oregano, and basil.
3. Bring to a boil, then reduce heat and simmer for 20 minutes until the quinoa is cooked and the vegetables are tender.
4. Stir in the chopped spinach and cook for an additional 5 minutes.
5. Serve warm.

Nutrition Info (per serving):
Calories: 180 Protein: 6g Fat: 3g Carbohydrates: 32g Fiber: 6g Sodium: 150mg
Servings: 4 **Cooking Time:** 30 minutes

7. Venison Broth

Ingredients:
- 1 pound venison stew meat, cubed
- 1 small onion, chopped
- 2 garlic cloves, minced
- 2 cups chopped carrots
- 2 cups chopped celery
- 8 cups low-sodium beef broth
- 1 teaspoon dried thyme
- 1 teaspoon dried rosemary

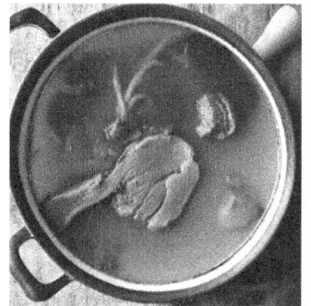

Instructions:
1. In a large pot, cook the venison stew meat over medium heat until browned.
2. Add the chopped onion and garlic, and sauté until softened, about 5 minutes.
3. Add the carrots, celery, beef broth, thyme, and rosemary.
4. Bring to a boil, then reduce heat and simmer for 1.5 hours until the venison is tender.
5. Serve warm.

Nutrition Info (per serving):
Calories: 180 Protein: 25g Fat: 4g Carbohydrates: 8g Fiber: 2g Sodium: 200mg
Servings: 6 **Cooking Time:** 1.5 hours

8. Duck and Ginger Broth

Ingredients:
- 1 pound duck breast, cooked and shredded
- 4 cups low-sodium chicken broth
- 1 small onion, chopped
- 2 garlic cloves, minced
- 1 tablespoon grated ginger
- 1 cup chopped bok choy

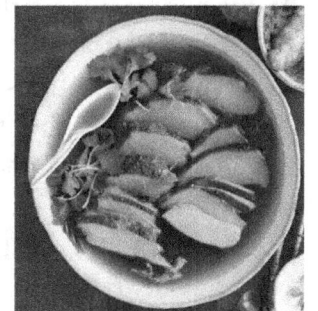

Instructions:
1. In a large pot, bring the chicken broth to a boil.
2. Add the chopped onion, garlic, and grated ginger, and simmer for 5 minutes.
3. Add the shredded duck and chopped bok choy.
4. Cook for an additional 10 minutes until the bok choy is tender.
5. Serve warm.

Nutrition Info (per serving):
- Calories: 160 Protein: 22g Fat: 6g Carbohydrates: 4g Fiber: 1g Sodium: 150mg

Servings: 4 **Cooking Time:** 20 minutes

9. Rabbit and Herb Soup

Ingredients:
- 1 pound rabbit meat, cubed
- 1 small onion, chopped
- 2 garlic cloves, minced
- 2 cups chopped carrots
- 2 cups chopped celery
- 4 cups low-sodium chicken broth
- 1 teaspoon dried thyme
- 1 teaspoon dried rosemary

Instructions:
1. In a large pot, cook the rabbit meat over medium heat until browned.
2. Add the chopped onion and garlic, and sauté until softened, about 5 minutes.
3. Add the carrots, celery, chicken broth, thyme, and rosemary.
4. Bring to a boil, then reduce heat and simmer for 1 hour until the rabbit is tender.
5. Serve warm.

Nutrition Info (per serving):
- Calories: 180 Protein: 25g
- Fat: 4g
- Carbohydrates: 8g
- Fiber: 2g
- Sodium: 150mg

Servings: 6 **Cooking Time:** 1 hour 15 minutes

10. Bison and Vegetable Broth

Ingredients:
- 1 pound ground bison
- 1 small onion, chopped
- 2 garlic cloves, minced
- 2 cups chopped carrots
- 2 cups chopped celery
- 4 cups low-sodium beef broth
- 1 teaspoon dried thyme

Instructions:
1. In a large pot, cook the ground bison over medium heat until browned.
2. Add the chopped onion and garlic, and sauté until softened, about 5 minutes.
3. Add the carrots, celery, and beef broth.
4. Bring to a boil, then reduce heat and simmer for 30 minutes until the vegetables are tender.
5. Stir in the thyme and cook for an additional 5 minutes.
6. Serve warm.

Nutrition Info (per serving):
Calories: 220 Protein: 28g Fat: 8g Carbohydrates: 8g Fiber: 2g Sodium: 200mg
Servings: 4 **Cooking Time:** 40 minutes

11. Spinach and Chicken Soup

Ingredients:
- 1 pound boneless, skinless chicken breasts, cooked and shredded
- 1 small onion, chopped
- 2 garlic cloves, minced
- 4 cups low-sodium chicken broth
- 2 cups chopped spinach
- 1 teaspoon dried oregano

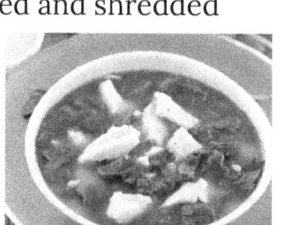

Instructions:
1. In a large pot, sauté the onion and garlic until softened, about 5 minutes.
2. Add the chicken broth and bring to a boil.
3. Reduce heat and simmer for 10 minutes.
4. Stir in the shredded chicken, chopped spinach, and oregano.
5. Cook for an additional 5 minutes until the spinach is wilted.
6. Serve warm.

Nutrition Info (per serving):
- Calories: 150 Protein: 25g Fat: 3g Carbohydrates: 4g Fiber: 1g
- Sodium: 150mg

Servings: 4 **Cooking Time:** 20 minutes

12. Pheasant Soup
Ingredients:
- 1 pound pheasant meat, cubed
- 1 small onion, chopped
- 2 garlic cloves, minced
- 2 cups chopped carrots
- 2 cups chopped celery
- 4 cups low-sodium chicken broth
- 1 teaspoon dried sage

Instructions:
1. In a large pot, cook the pheasant meat over medium heat until browned.
2. Add the chopped onion and garlic, and sauté until softened, about 5 minutes.
3. Add the carrots, celery, chicken broth, and sage.
4. Bring to a boil, then reduce heat and simmer for 1 hour until the pheasant is tender.
5. Serve warm.

Nutrition Info (per serving):
Calories: 180 Protein: 25g Fat: 4g Carbohydrates: 8g Fiber: 2g Sodium: 150mg
Servings: 6 **Cooking Time:** 1 hour 15 minutes

13. Soft Cod Soup
Ingredients:
- 1 pound cod fillets, cubed
- 1 small onion, chopped
- 2 garlic cloves, minced
- 2 cups chopped leeks
- 4 cups low-sodium fish broth
- 1 teaspoon dried dill

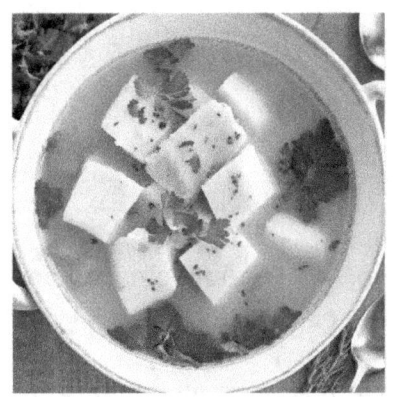

Instructions:
1. In a large pot, sauté the onion, garlic, and leeks until softened, about 5 minutes.
2. Add the fish broth and bring to a boil.
3. Reduce heat and simmer for 10 minutes.
4. Stir in the cubed cod and dill.
5. Cook for an additional 5-7 minutes until the cod is cooked through.
6. Serve warm.

Nutrition Info (per serving):
- Calories: 140 Protein: 24g Fat: 2g Carbohydrates: 6g Fiber: 2g
- Sodium: 150mg

Servings: 4 **Cooking Time:** 25 minutes

14. Smooth Asparagus and Turkey Soup

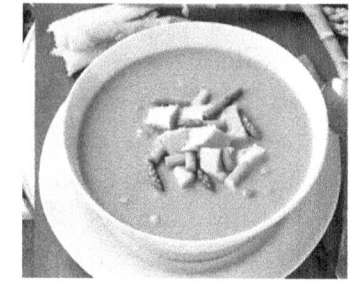

Ingredients:
- 1 pound cooked turkey breast, shredded
- 1 small onion, chopped
- 2 garlic cloves, minced
- 2 cups chopped asparagus
- 4 cups low-sodium chicken broth
- 1/2 cup low-fat Greek yogurt

Instructions:
1. In a large pot, sauté the onion and garlic until softened, about 5 minutes.
2. Add the chopped asparagus and chicken broth, and bring to a boil.
3. Reduce heat and simmer for 10 minutes.
4. Use an immersion blender to blend the soup until smooth.
5. Stir in the shredded turkey and Greek yogurt.
6. Cook for an additional 5 minutes.
7. Serve warm.

Nutrition Info (per serving):
Calories: 160 Protein: 25g Fat: 3g Carbohydrates: 6g Fiber: 2g Sodium: 150mg
Servings: 4 **Cooking Time:** 25 minutes

15. Parsnip and Pork Soup

Ingredients:
- 1 pound pork tenderloin, cubed
- 1 small onion, chopped
- 2 garlic cloves, minced
- 2 cups chopped parsnips
- 4 cups low-sodium chicken broth
- 1 teaspoon dried thyme

Instructions:
1. In a large pot, cook the pork tenderloin over medium heat until browned.
2. Add the chopped onion and garlic, and sauté until softened, about 5 minutes.
3. Add the chopped parsnips and chicken broth.
4. Bring to a boil, then reduce heat and simmer for 30 minutes until the parsnips are tender.
5. Stir in the thyme and cook for an additional 5 minutes.
6. Serve warm.

Nutrition Info (per serving):
- Calories: 200 Protein: 25g Fat: 5g Carbohydrates: 12g Fiber: 4g
- Sodium: 150mg

Servings: 4 **Cooking Time:** 40 minutes

16. Cauliflower and Cod Stew
Ingredients:
- 1 pound cod fillets, cubed
- 1 small onion, chopped
- 2 garlic cloves, minced
- 2 cups cauliflower florets
- 4 cups low-sodium chicken broth
- 1 teaspoon dried basil

Instructions:
1. In a large pot, sauté the onion and garlic until softened, about 5 minutes.
2. Add the cauliflower florets and chicken broth, and bring to a boil.
3. Reduce heat and simmer for 10 minutes.
4. Stir in the cubed cod and basil.
5. Cook for an additional 5-7 minutes until the cod is cooked through and the cauliflower is tender.
6. Serve warm.

Nutrition Info (per serving):
- Calories: 150 Protein: 24g Fat: 2g Carbohydrates: 6g Fiber: 3g
- Sodium: 150mg

Servings: 4 **Cooking Time:** 25 minutes

17. Tender Goat Meat Stew
Ingredients:
- 1 pound goat meat, cubed
- 1 small onion, chopped
- 2 garlic cloves, minced
- 2 cups chopped carrots
- 2 cups chopped potatoes
- 4 cups low-sodium beef broth
- 1 teaspoon dried rosemary

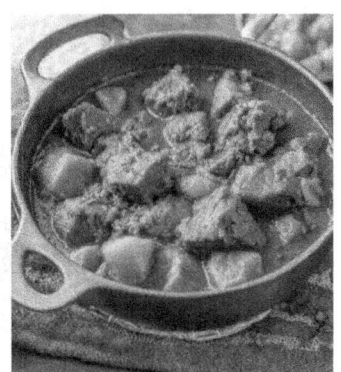

Instructions:
1. In a large pot, cook the goat meat over medium heat until browned.
2. Add the chopped onion and garlic, and sauté until softened, about 5 minutes.
3. Add the carrots, potatoes, beef broth, and rosemary.
4. Bring to a boil, then reduce heat and simmer for 1.5 hours until the goat meat is tender.
5. Serve warm.

Nutrition Info (per serving):
Calories: 220 Protein: 25g Fat: 8g Carbohydrates: 12g Fiber: 3g
- Sodium: 200mg

Servings: 6 **Cooking Time:** 1.5 hours

18. Chicken Gizzard Soup

Ingredients:
- 1 pound chicken gizzards, cleaned and chopped
- 1 small onion, chopped
- 2 garlic cloves, minced
- 2 cups chopped carrots
- 2 cups chopped celery
- 4 cups low-sodium chicken broth
- 1 teaspoon dried thyme

Instructions:
1. In a large pot, cook the chicken gizzards over medium heat until browned.
2. Add the chopped onion and garlic, and sauté until softened, about 5 minutes.
3. Add the carrots, celery, chicken broth, and thyme.
4. Bring to a boil, then reduce heat and simmer for 1 hour until the gizzards are tender.
5. Serve warm.

Nutrition Info (per serving):
- Calories: 180
- Protein: 25g
- Fat: 4g
- Carbohydrates: 8g
- Fiber: 2g
- Sodium: 150mg

Servings: 6 **Cooking Time:** 1 hour 15 minutes

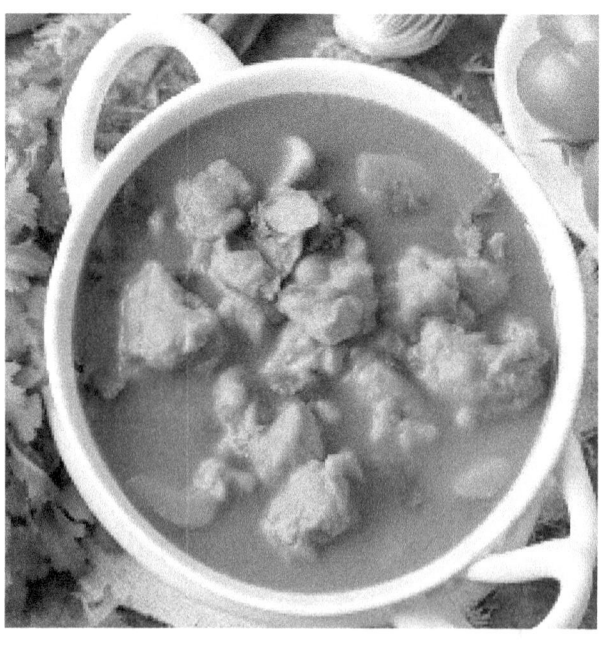

Desserts & Snacks

1. Coconut Milk Rice Pudding
Ingredients:
- 1 cup cooked white rice
- 1 cup light coconut milk
- 1/4 cup water
- 2 tablespoons honey or maple syrup
- 1/2 teaspoon vanilla extract
- 1/4 teaspoon ground cinnamon

Instructions:
1. In a saucepan, combine the cooked rice, coconut milk, water, honey or maple syrup, and cinnamon.
2. Cook over medium heat, stirring frequently, until the mixture thickens, about 10-15 minutes.
3. Remove from heat and stir in the vanilla extract.
4. Serve warm or chilled.

Nutrition Info (per serving):
- Calories: 120
- Protein: 2g
- Fat: 4g
- Carbohydrates: 20g
- Fiber: 1g
- Sodium: 20mg

Servings: 4 **Cooking Time:** 15 minutes

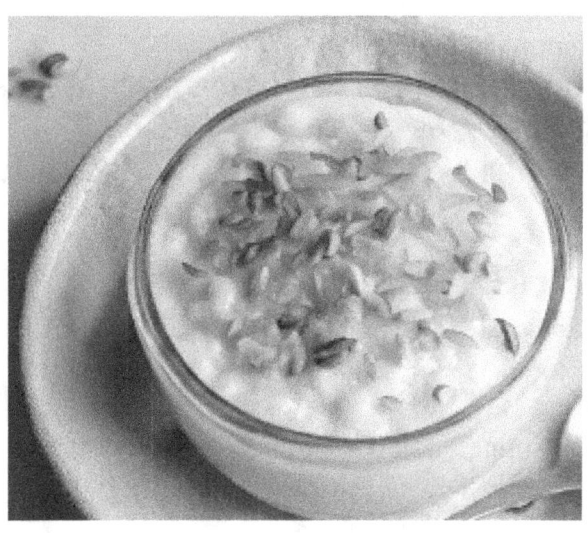

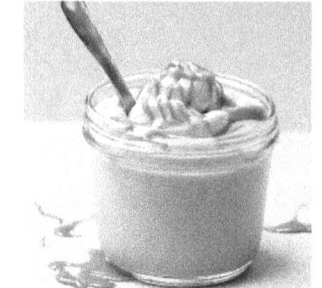

2. Caramel Protein Mousse

Ingredients:
- 1 cup low-fat Greek yogurt
- 1 scoop caramel-flavored protein powder
- 1 tablespoon caramel sauce (sugar-free if preferred)
- 1/2 teaspoon vanilla extract

Instructions:
1. In a bowl, combine the Greek yogurt, protein powder, caramel sauce, and vanilla extract.
2. Mix until smooth and well combined.
3. Chill in the refrigerator for at least 1 hour before serving.

Nutrition Info (per serving):
- Calories: 130 Protein: 20g Fat: 1g Carbohydrates: 10g
- Fiber: 0g
- Sodium: 100mg

Servings: 2 **Cooking Time:** 5 minutes (plus 1 hour chilling time)

3. Peaches and Cream Protein Smoothie

Ingredients:
- 1 cup unsweetened almond milk
- 1 cup frozen peach slices
- 1 scoop vanilla protein powder
- 1/2 teaspoon vanilla extract

Instructions:
1. Place all ingredients in a blender.
2. Blend until smooth.
3. Serve immediately.

Nutrition Info (per serving):
- Calories: 150
- Protein: 20g
- Fat: 3g
- Carbohydrates: 15g
- Fiber: 3g
- Sodium: 150mg

Servings: 2 **Cooking Time:** 5 minutes

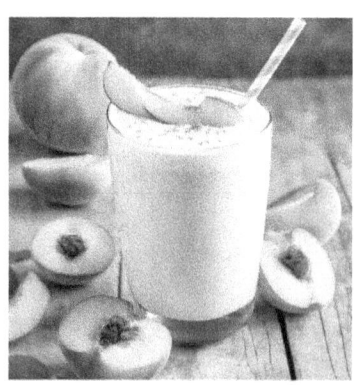

4. Soft Baked Protein Apple Slices

Ingredients:
- 2 large apples, peeled, cored, and sliced
- 1 scoop vanilla protein powder
- 1 tablespoon honey or maple syrup
- 1 teaspoon ground cinnamon

Instructions:
1. Preheat the oven to 350°F (175°C).
2. In a bowl, combine the apple slices, protein powder, honey or maple syrup, and cinnamon.
3. Toss until the apple slices are evenly coated.
4. Spread the apple slices on a baking sheet lined with parchment paper.
5. Bake for 20 minutes, or until the apples are tender.
6. Serve warm.

Nutrition Info (per serving):
- Calories: 100
- Protein: 10g
- Fat: 0g
- Carbohydrates: 22g
- Fiber: 4g
- Sodium: 30mg

Servings: 4 **Cooking Time:** 20 minutes

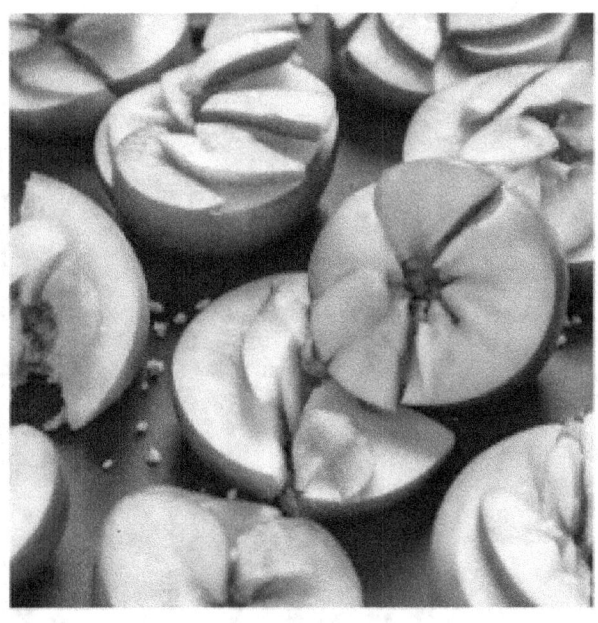

5. Chocolate Hazelnut Spread

Ingredients:
- 1 cup raw hazelnuts
- 2 tablespoons cocoa powder
- 1/4 cup powdered sugar or sugar substitute
- 1/4 cup skim milk
- 1 teaspoon vanilla extract

Instructions:
1. Preheat the oven to 350°F (175°C).
2. Spread the hazelnuts on a baking sheet and roast for 10-12 minutes.
3. Allow the hazelnuts to cool, then rub them with a kitchen towel to remove the skins.
4. In a food processor, blend the hazelnuts until they form a smooth butter.
5. Add the cocoa powder, powdered sugar, skim milk, and vanilla extract.
6. Blend until smooth and well combined.
7. Store in an airtight container in the refrigerator.

Nutrition Info (per serving):
- Calories: 90
- Protein: 2g
- Fat: 7g
- Carbohydrates: 7g
- Fiber: 1g
- Sodium: 10mg

Servings: 8 **Cooking Time:** 15 minutes

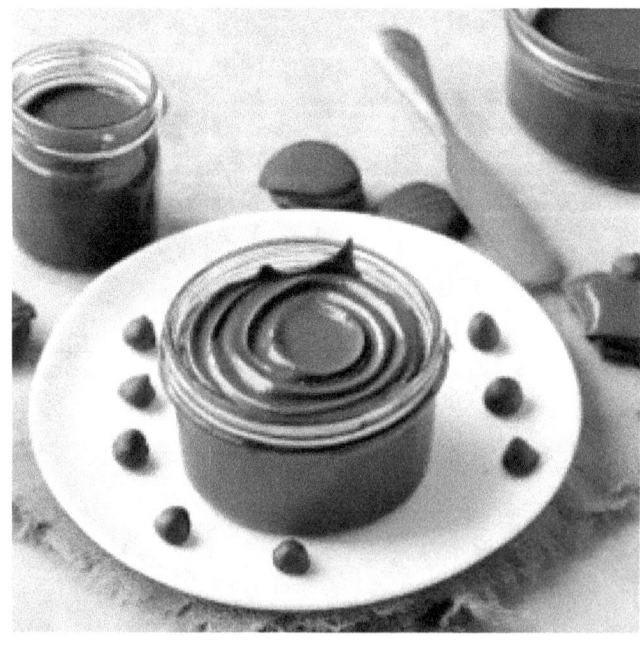

6. Maple Almond Protein Custard

Ingredients:
- 1 cup unsweetened almond milk
- 1 scoop vanilla protein powder
- 2 tablespoons maple syrup
- 1/2 teaspoon almond extract
- 2 large eggs

Instructions:
1. Preheat the oven to 325°F (160°C).
2. In a bowl, whisk together the almond milk, protein powder, maple syrup, almond extract, and eggs until smooth.
3. Pour the mixture into ramekins.
4. Place the ramekins in a baking dish and add hot water to the dish until it reaches halfway up the sides of the ramekins.
5. Bake for 30-35 minutes, or until the custard is set.
6. Allow to cool before serving.

Nutrition Info (per serving):
- Calories: 120
- Protein: 12g
- Fat: 4g
- Carbohydrates: 10g
- Fiber: 1g
- Sodium: 80mg

Servings: 4 **Cooking Time:** 35 minutes

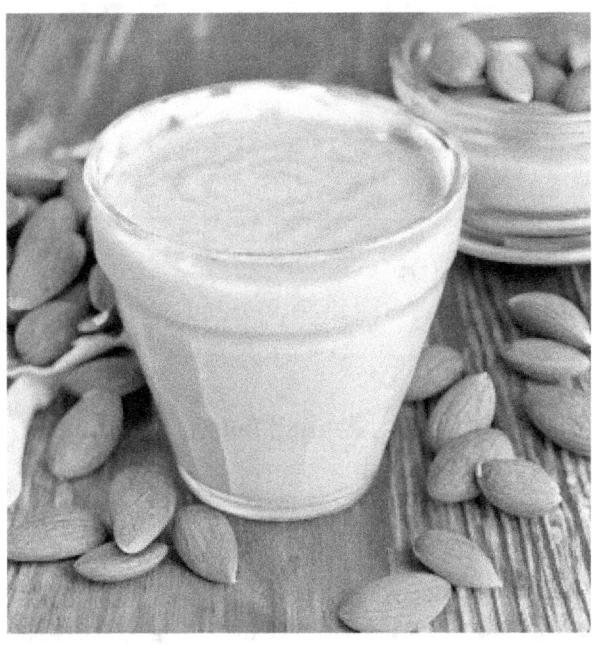

7. Pumpkin Spice Soft Cookies

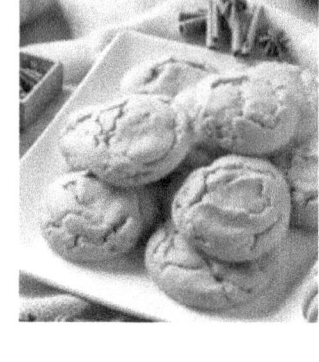

Ingredients:
- 1 cup pumpkin puree
- 1/2 cup oat flour
- 1/4 cup vanilla protein powder
- 1/4 cup honey or maple syrup
- 1 teaspoon pumpkin pie spice
- 1/2 teaspoon baking soda

Instructions:
1. Preheat the oven to 350°F (175°C).
2. In a bowl, combine the pumpkin puree, oat flour, protein powder, honey or maple syrup, pumpkin pie spice, and baking soda.
3. Mix until well combined.
4. Drop spoonfuls of the dough onto a baking sheet lined with parchment paper.
5. Bake for 10-12 minutes, or until the cookies are set.
6. Allow to cool before serving.

Nutrition Info (per serving):
Calories: 80 Protein: 5g Fat: 1g Carbohydrates: 14g Fiber: 2g
- Sodium: 60mg

Servings: 12 **Cooking Time:** 12 minutes

8. Soft Carrot Cake Squares

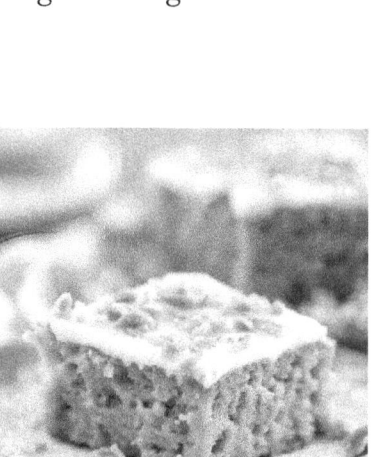

Ingredients:
- 1 cup grated carrots
- 1/2 cup oat flour
- 1/4 cup vanilla protein powder
- 1/4 cup honey or maple syrup
- 2 large eggs
- 1 teaspoon ground cinnamon
- 1/2 teaspoon baking soda

Instructions:
1. Preheat the oven to 350°F (175°C).
2. In a bowl, combine the grated carrots, oat flour, protein powder, honey or maple syrup, eggs, cinnamon, and baking soda.
3. Mix until well combined.
4. Pour the batter into a greased 8x8-inch baking dish.
5. Bake for 20-25 minutes, or until a toothpick inserted into the center comes out clean.
6. Allow to cool before cutting into squares.

Nutrition Info (per serving):
Calories: 90 Protein: 6g Fat: 2g Carbohydrates: 12g Fiber: 2g Sodium: 70mg
Servings: 9 **Cooking Time:** 25 minutes

9. Protein Flan

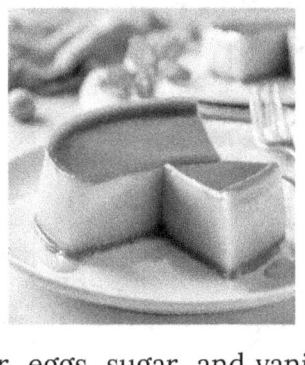

Ingredients:
- 1 cup low-fat milk
- 1 scoop vanilla protein powder
- 3 large eggs
- 1/4 cup sugar or sugar substitute
- 1 teaspoon vanilla extract

Instructions:
1. Preheat the oven to 325°F (160°C).
2. In a bowl, whisk together the milk, protein powder, eggs, sugar, and vanilla extract until smooth.
3. Pour the mixture into ramekins.
4. Place the ramekins in a baking dish and add hot water to the dish until it reaches halfway up the sides of the ramekins.
5. Bake for 30-35 minutes, or until the flan is set.
6. Allow to cool before serving.

Nutrition Info (per serving):
Calories: 100 Protein: 10g Fat: 3g Carbohydrates: 10g Fiber: 0g Sodium: 60mg
Servings: 4 **Cooking Time:** 35 minutes

10. Low-fat Tiramisu

Ingredients:
- 1 cup low-fat ricotta cheese
- 1/2 cup low-fat Greek yogurt
- 1/4 cup brewed espresso, cooled
- 2 tablespoons honey or sugar substitute
- 1/2 teaspoon vanilla extract
- 1/4 cup unsweetened cocoa powder
- 4 whole-wheat ladyfinger cookies

Instructions:
1. In a bowl, combine the ricotta cheese, Greek yogurt, honey, and vanilla extract. Mix until smooth.
2. Dip each ladyfinger cookie in the cooled espresso and layer them in a small dish.
3. Spread half of the ricotta mixture over the ladyfingers.
4. Repeat with another layer of dipped ladyfingers and the remaining ricotta mixture.
5. Dust the top with cocoa powder.
6. Chill in the refrigerator for at least 1 hour before serving.

Nutrition Info (per serving):
Calories: 150 Protein: 10g Fat: 4g Carbohydrates: 20g Fiber: 2g Sodium: 80mg
Servings: 4 **Cooking Time:** 10 minutes (plus 1 hour chilling time)

11. Creamy Banana Soft Serve

Ingredients:
- 2 ripe bananas, sliced and frozen
- 1/4 cup low-fat Greek yogurt
- 1 teaspoon vanilla extract

Instructions:
1. Place the frozen banana slices in a food processor or blender.
2. Add the Greek yogurt and vanilla extract.
3. Blend until smooth and creamy.
4. Serve immediately.

Nutrition Info (per serving):
- Calories: 90
- Protein: 3g
- Fat: 0g
- Carbohydrates: 21g
- Fiber: 3g
- Sodium: 10mg

Servings: 2 **Cooking Time:** 5 minutes

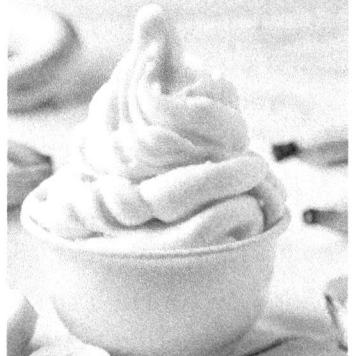

12. Cacao Nib Protein Yogurt

Ingredients:
- 1 cup low-fat Greek yogurt
- 1 scoop chocolate protein powder
- 1 tablespoon cacao nibs
- 1 teaspoon honey or agave syrup (optional)

Instructions:
1. In a bowl, combine the Greek yogurt and chocolate protein powder. Mix until smooth.
2. Stir in the cacao nibs.
3. Drizzle with honey or agave syrup if desired.
4. Serve immediately.

Nutrition Info (per serving):
- Calories: 160
- Protein: 20g
- Fat: 3g
- Carbohydrates: 15g
- Fiber: 2g
- Sodium: 80mg

Servings: 1 **Cooking Time:** 5 minutes

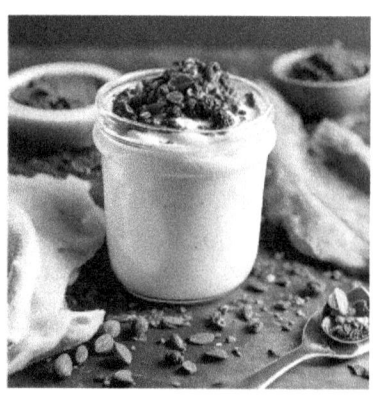

13. Fluffy Protein Pancakes

Ingredients:
- 1/2 cup oat flour
- 1 scoop vanilla protein powder
- 1/2 teaspoon baking powder
- 1/2 cup unsweetened almond milk
- 1 large egg
- 1/2 teaspoon vanilla extract
- Non-stick cooking spray

Instructions:
1. In a bowl, combine the oat flour, protein powder, and baking powder.
2. Add the almond milk, egg, and vanilla extract. Mix until smooth.
3. Heat a non-stick skillet over medium heat and spray with cooking spray.
4. Pour small amounts of the batter into the skillet to form pancakes.
5. Cook until bubbles form on the surface, then flip and cook until golden brown, about 2-3 minutes per side.
6. Serve warm.

Nutrition Info (per serving):
- Calories: 180
- Protein: 15g
- Fat: 5g
- Carbohydrates: 20g
- Fiber: 3g
- Sodium: 150mg

Servings: 2 **Cooking Time:** 10 minutes

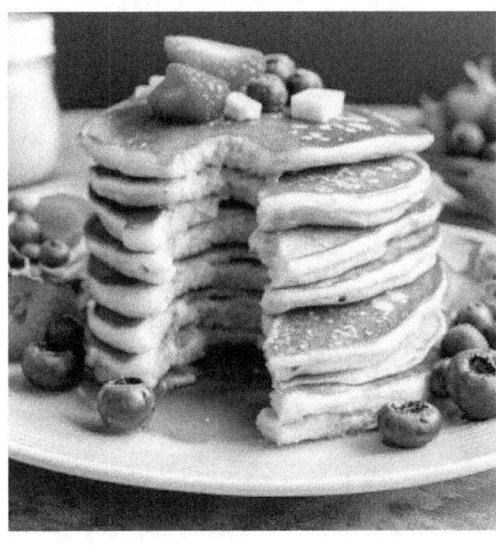

8-Week Meal Plan.

Week 1: Clear Liquids
Breakfast:
- Homemade Chicken Broth

Lunch:
- Vegetable Broth

Snack:
- White Grape Juice

Dinner:
- Beef Broth

Week 2: Clear Liquids
Breakfast:
- Mint Tea

Lunch:
- Clear Iced Tea

Snack:
- Japanese Clear Soup

Dinner:
- Chicken Gelatin

Week 3: Full Liquids
Breakfast:
- Smooth Cream of Wheat

Lunch:
- Blended Pumpkin Soup

Snack:
- Banana Smoothie

Dinner:
- Mashed Potato Soup

Week 4: Full Liquids
Breakfast:
- Avocado Smoothie

Lunch:
- Pea Soup

Snack:
- Yogurt Smoothie

Dinner:
- Pear & Ricotta Puree

Week 5: Pureed Foods
Breakfast:
- Malted Milk Drink

Lunch:
- Shrimp Scampi Puree

Snack:
- Rice Congee

Dinner:
- Egg Custard

Week 6: Pureed Foods
Breakfast:
- Strained Cream Soups

Lunch:
- Honeydew Melon Juice

Snack:
- Soft Cheesecake

Dinner:
- Baba Ghanoush

Week 7: Soft Foods
Breakfast:
- Greek Yogurt with Mashed Berries

Lunch:
- Soft Cooked Chicken Thighs

Snack:
- Protein Enriched Apple Smoothie

Dinner:
- Pureed White Fish

Week 8: Soft Foods
Breakfast:
- Fluffy Egg Whites

Lunch:
- Ground Turkey Soup

Snack:
- Creamy Banana Soft Serve

Dinner:
- Soft Salmon Mousse

Sample Days for Week 9 and Beyond (Transition to Regular Foods)

Day 1Breakfast:
- Peaches and Cream Protein Smoothie

Lunch:
- Chicken Liver Pate

Snack:
- Protein Flan

Dinner:
- Soft Meatballs in Tomato Sauce

Day 2Breakfast:
- Fluffy Protein Pancakes

Lunch:
- Turkey and Sage Soup

Snack:
- Cacao Nib Protein Yogurt

Dinner:
- Mild Mackerel Puree

Day 3Breakfast:
- Low-fat Tiramisu

Lunch:
- Rabbit and Herb Soup

Snack:
- Caramel Protein Mousse

Dinner:
- Tender Goat Meat Stew

Weekly Breakdown

Weeks 1-2: Clear Liquids
Focus on hydration and basic nutrients from clear broths, juices, and teas.

Weeks 3-4: Full Liquids
Introduce smooth, protein-rich liquids and soups to increase nutrient intake.

Weeks 5-6: Pureed Foods
Begin incorporating smooth purees of protein and vegetables to ease digestion.

Weeks 7-8: Soft Foods
Transition to soft, easy-to-chew proteins and vegetables.

Weeks 9 and Beyond: Regular Foods
Gradually return to more solid foods while maintaining a focus on high protein, low sugar, and low-fat meals.

MONTH.1.

Weight Loss Tracker

Starting Weight

Goal Weight

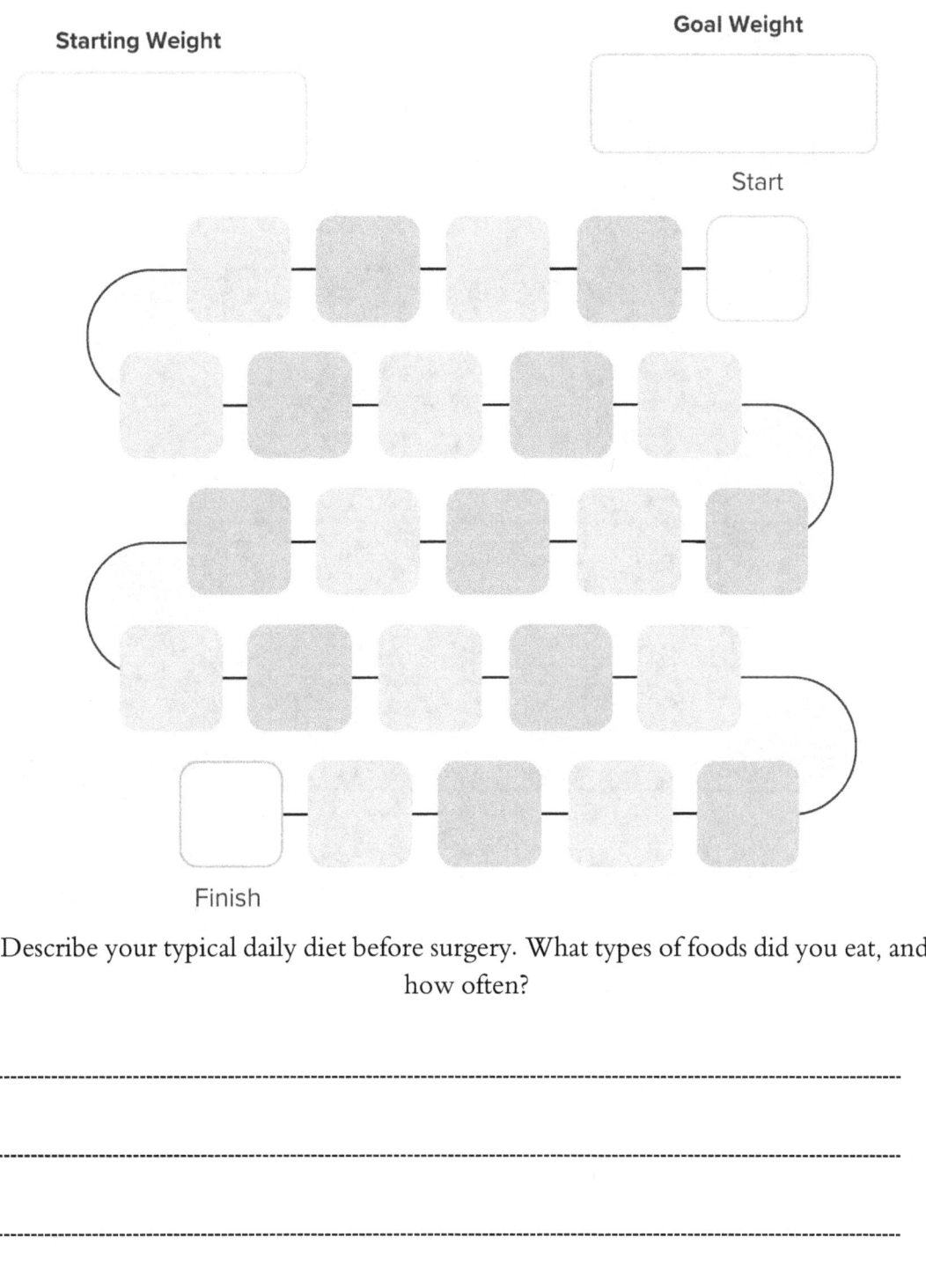

Describe your typical daily diet before surgery. What types of foods did you eat, and how often?

MONTH.2.

Weight Loss Tracker

Starting Weight

Goal Weight

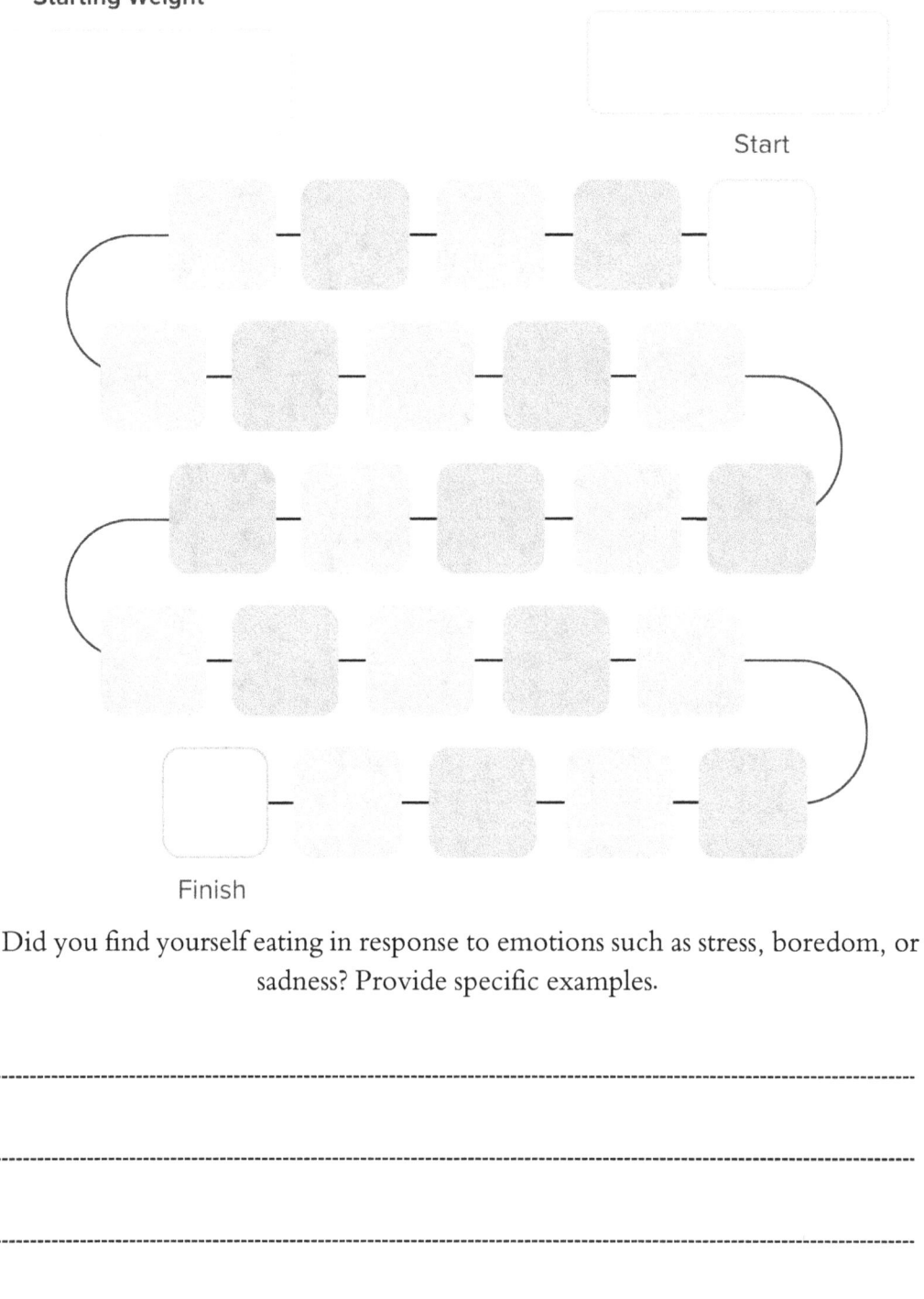

Start

Finish

Did you find yourself eating in response to emotions such as stress, boredom, or sadness? Provide specific examples.

MONTH.3.

Weight Loss Tracker

Starting Weight

Goal Weight

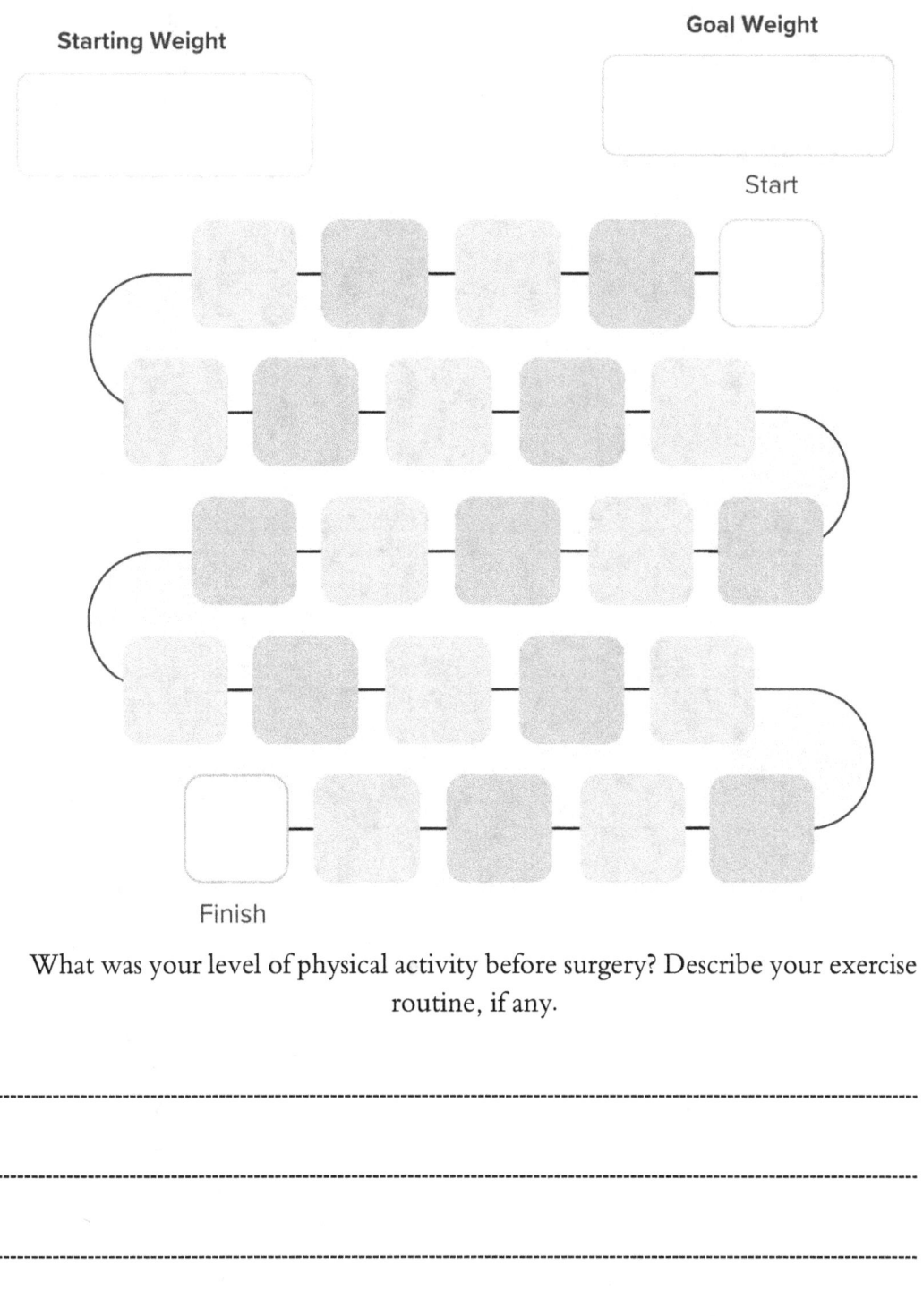

Start

Finish

What was your level of physical activity before surgery? Describe your exercise routine, if any.

MONTH.4.

Weight Loss Tracker

Starting Weight **Goal Weight**

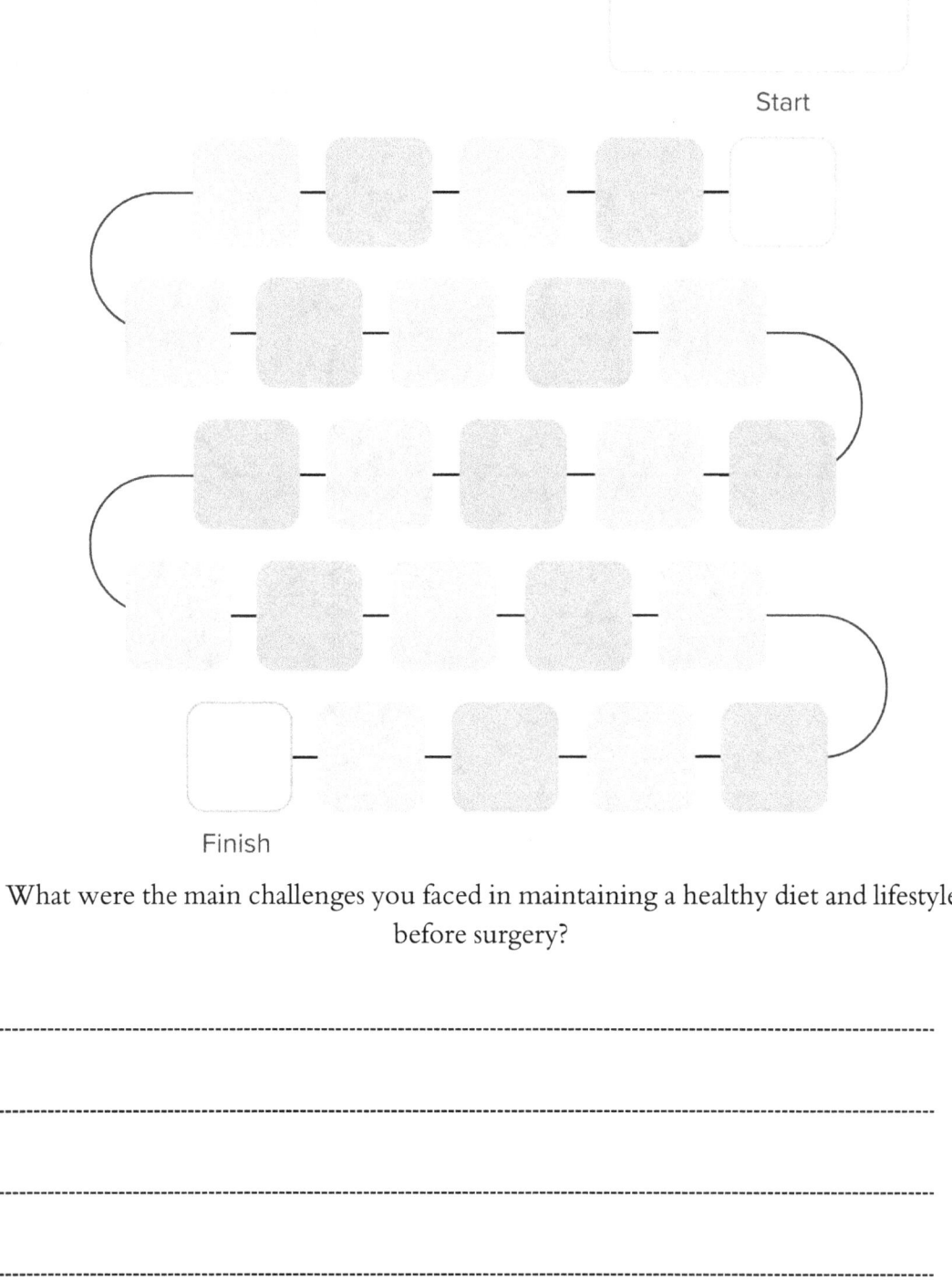

What were the main challenges you faced in maintaining a healthy diet and lifestyle before surgery?

MONTH.5.
Weight Loss Tracker

Starting Weight

Goal Weight

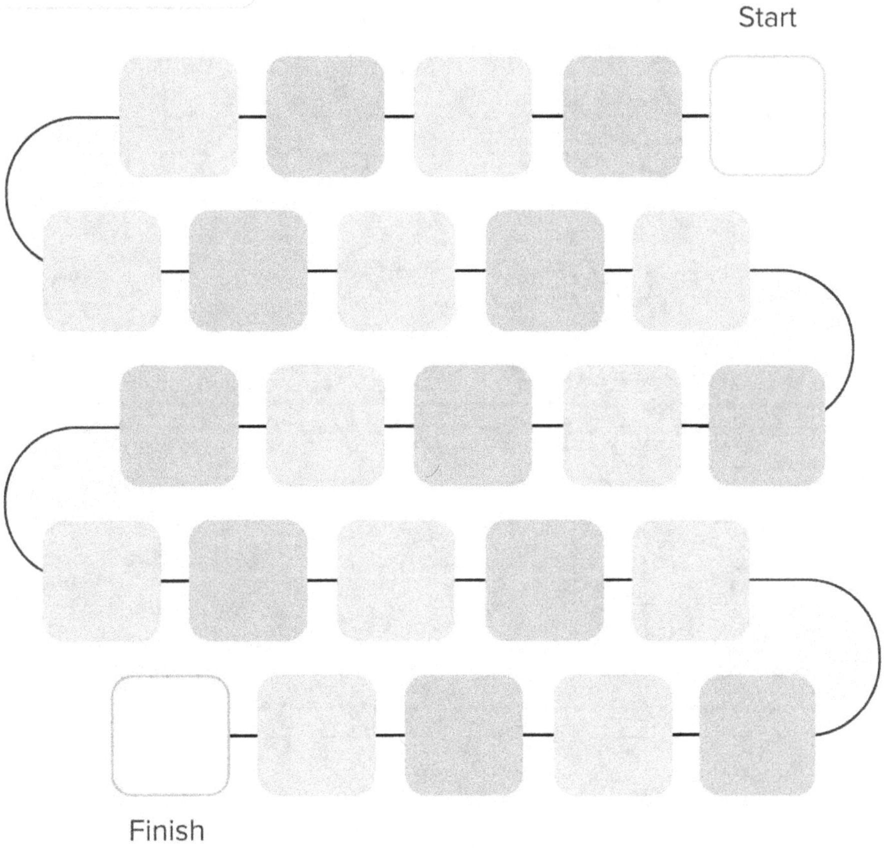

Start

Finish

What immediate changes have you noticed in your appetite and eating habits since the surgery?

MONTH.6.

Weight Loss Tracker

Starting Weight   **Goal Weight**

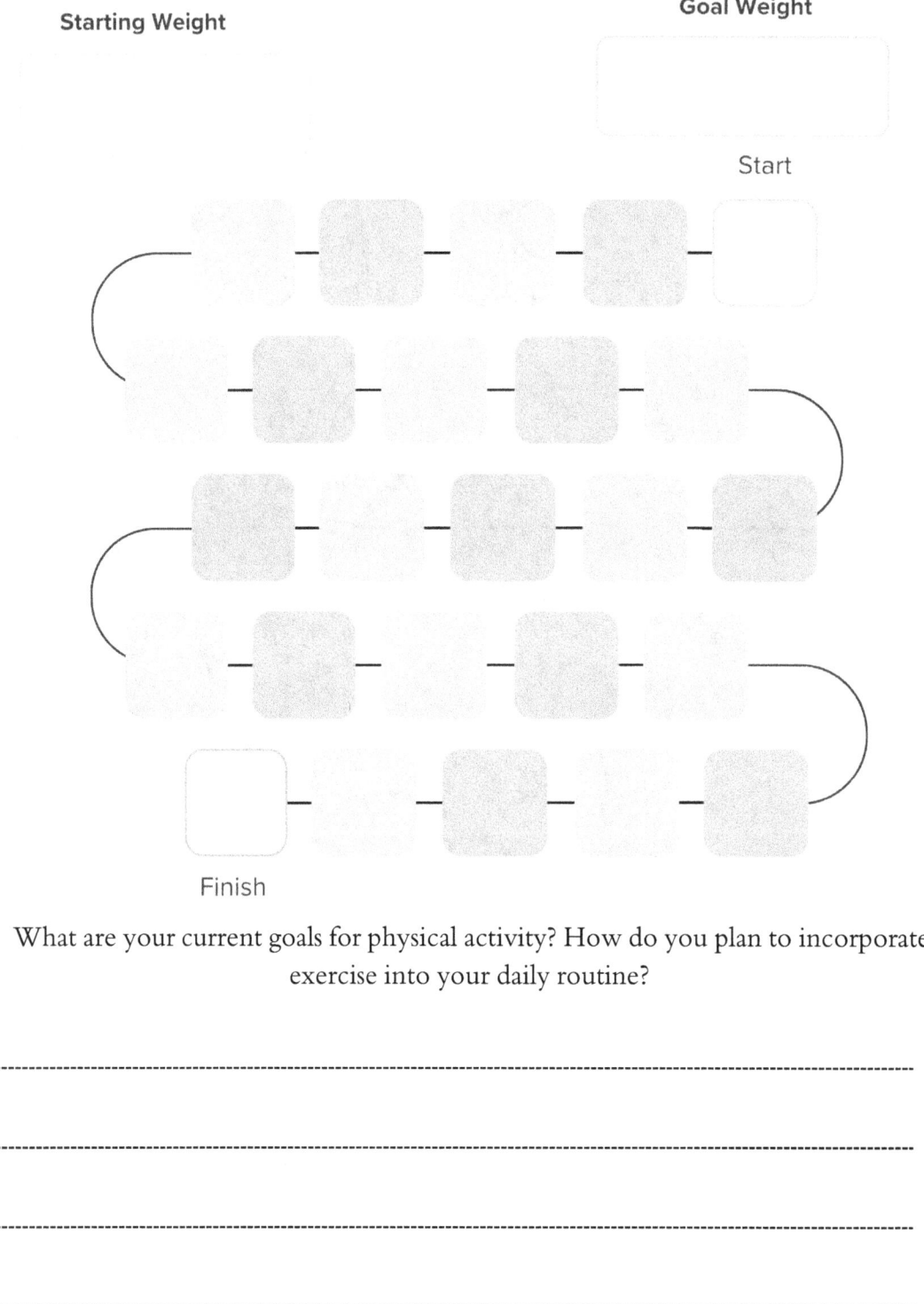

Start

Finish

What are your current goals for physical activity? How do you plan to incorporate exercise into your daily routine?

MONTH.7.

Weight Loss Tracker

Starting Weight

Goal Weight

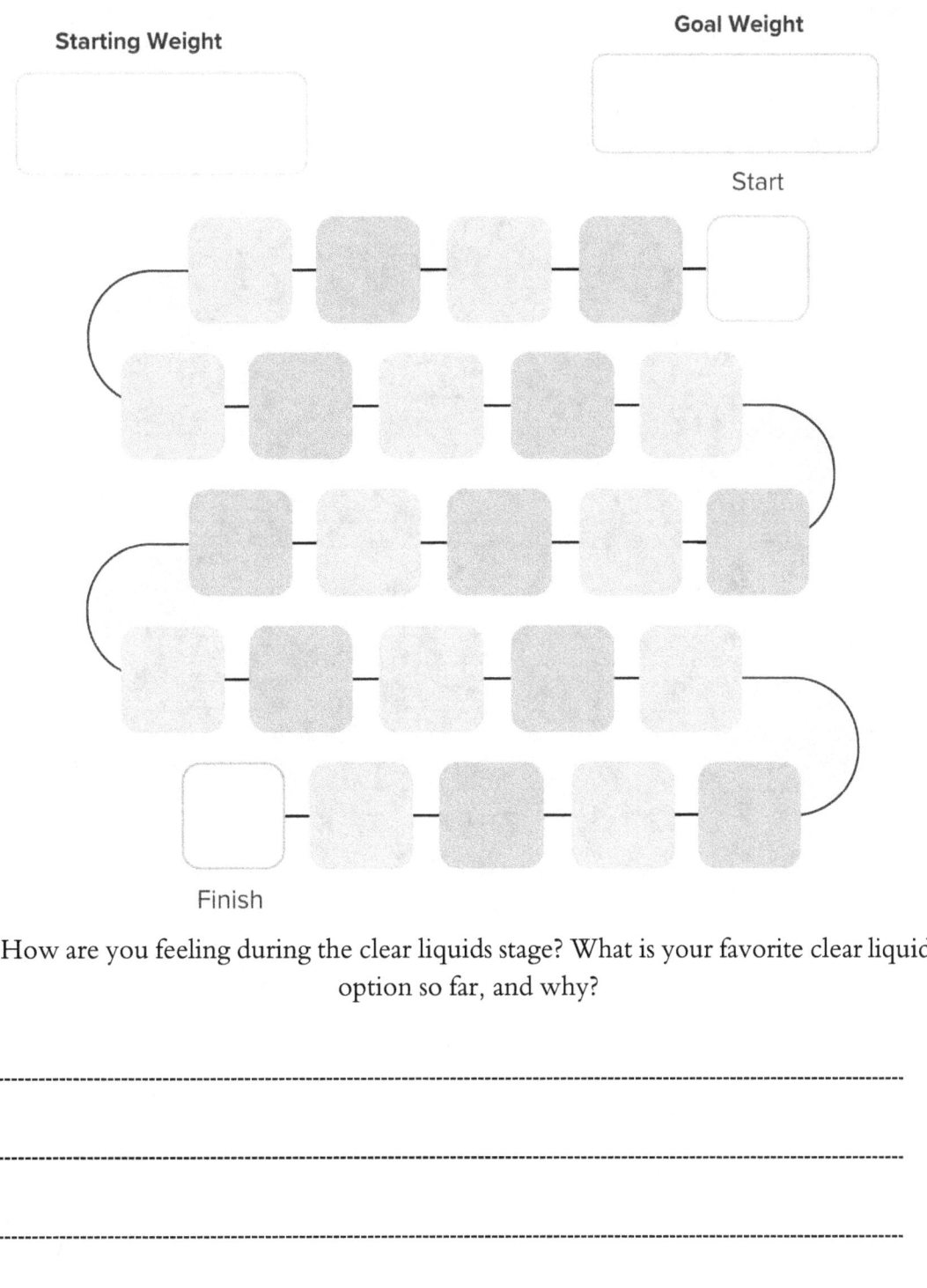

Start

Finish

How are you feeling during the clear liquids stage? What is your favorite clear liquid option so far, and why?

MONTH.8.
Weight Loss Tracker

Starting Weight   **Goal Weight**

Start

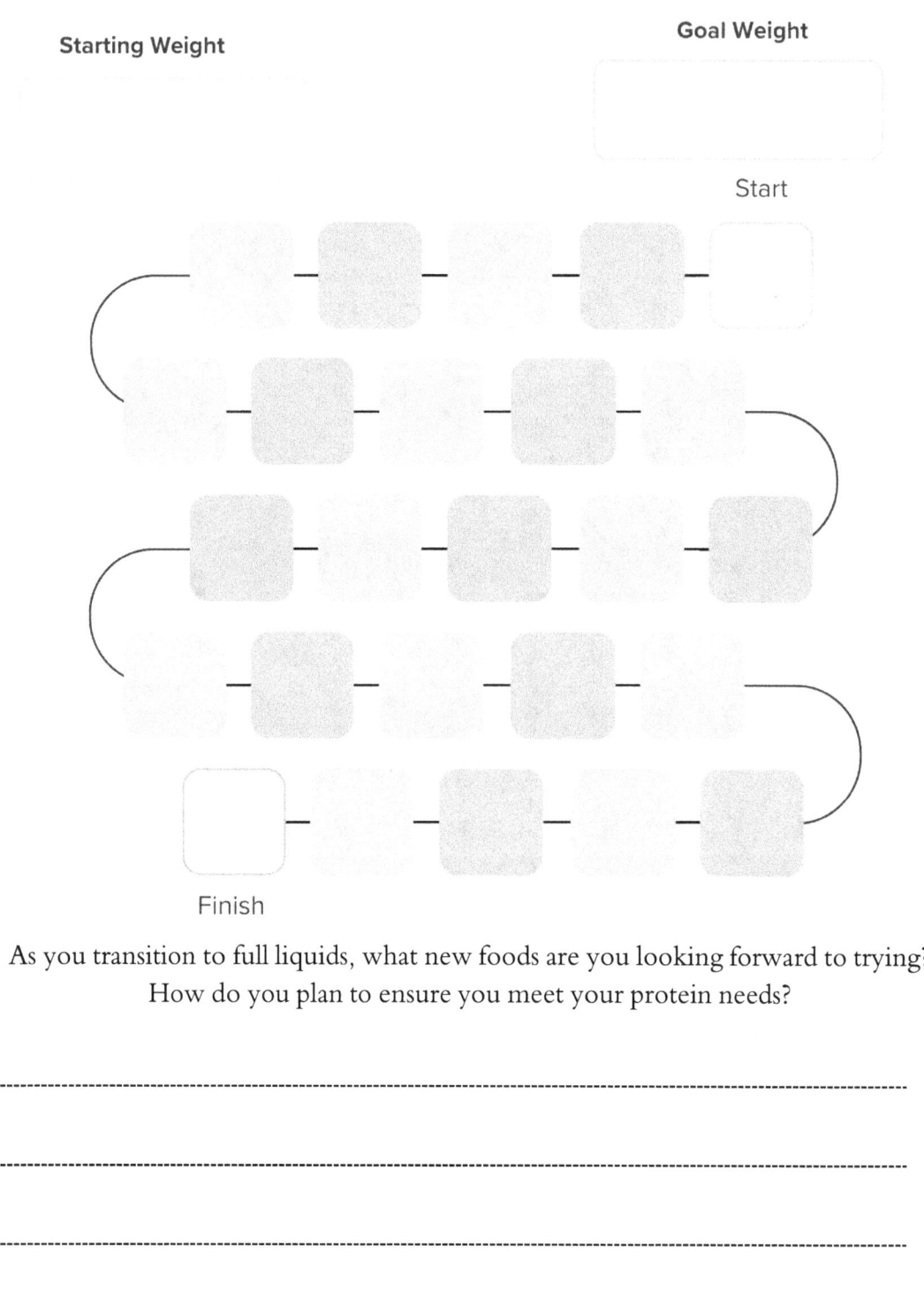

Finish

As you transition to full liquids, what new foods are you looking forward to trying? How do you plan to ensure you meet your protein needs?

MONTH.9.
Weight Loss Tracker

Starting Weight

Goal Weight

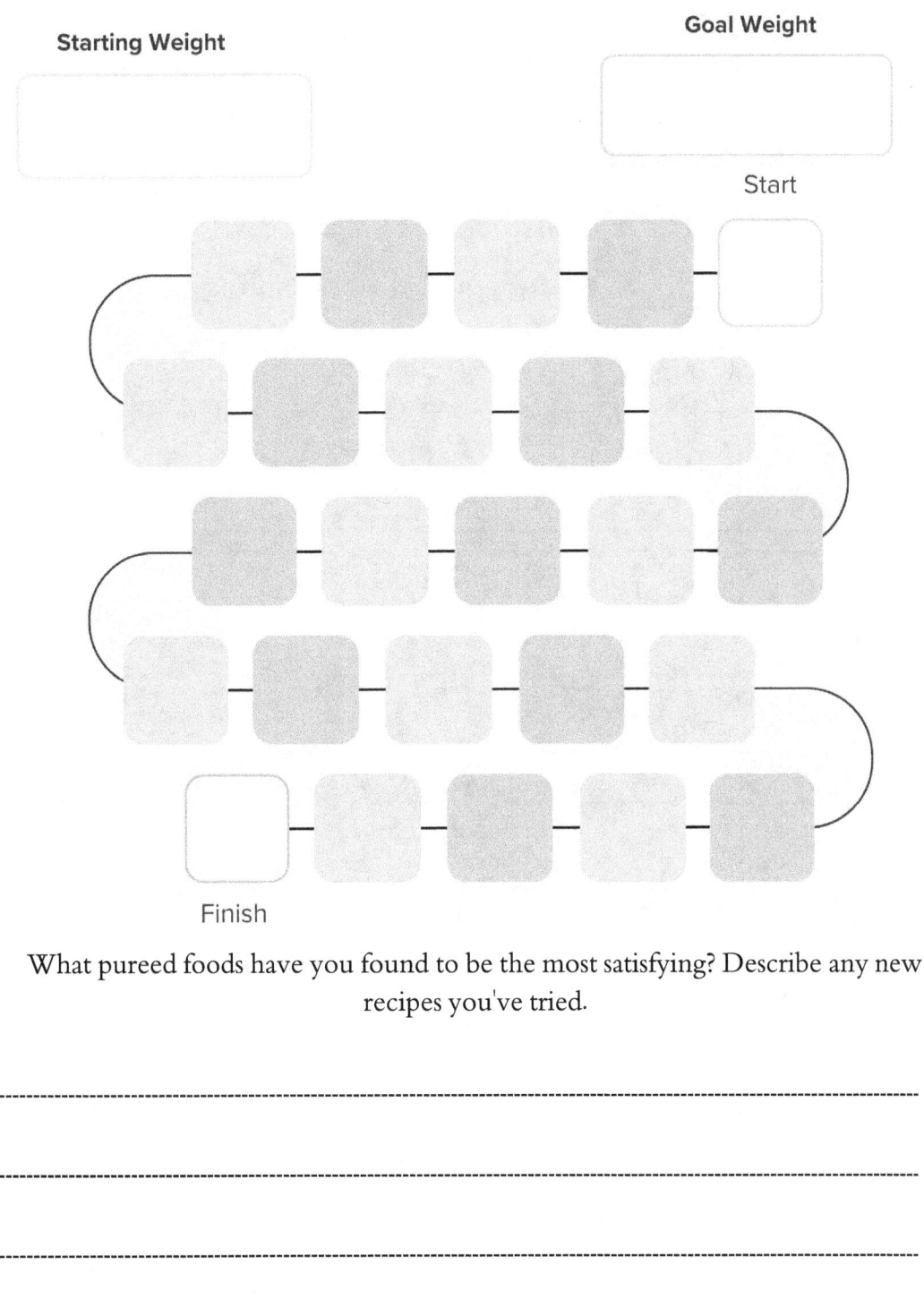

What pureed foods have you found to be the most satisfying? Describe any new recipes you've tried.

MONTH.10.
Weight Loss Tracker

Starting Weight

Goal Weight

Start

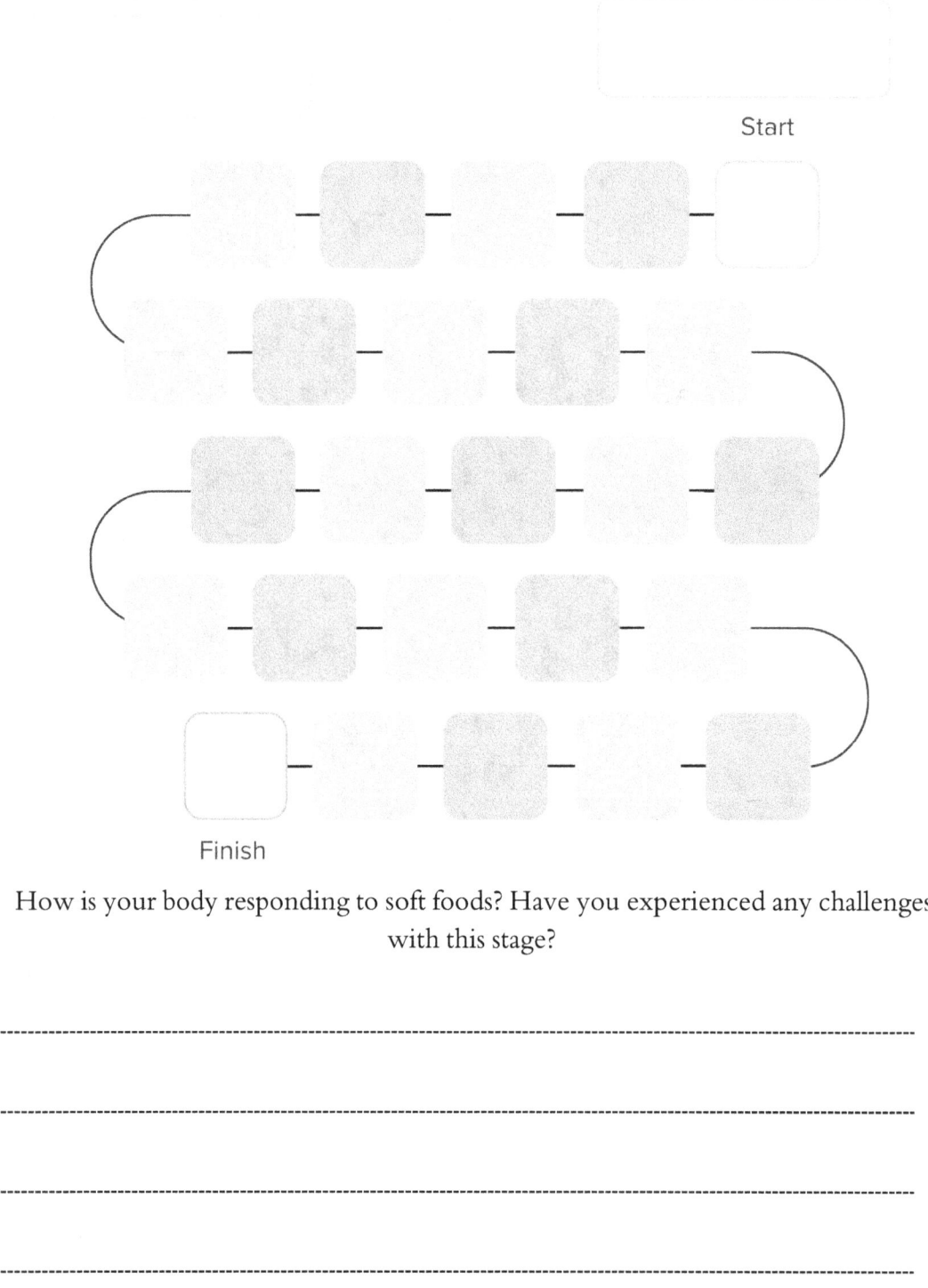

Finish

How is your body responding to soft foods? Have you experienced any challenges with this stage?

MONTH.11.

Weight Loss Tracker

Starting Weight

Goal Weight

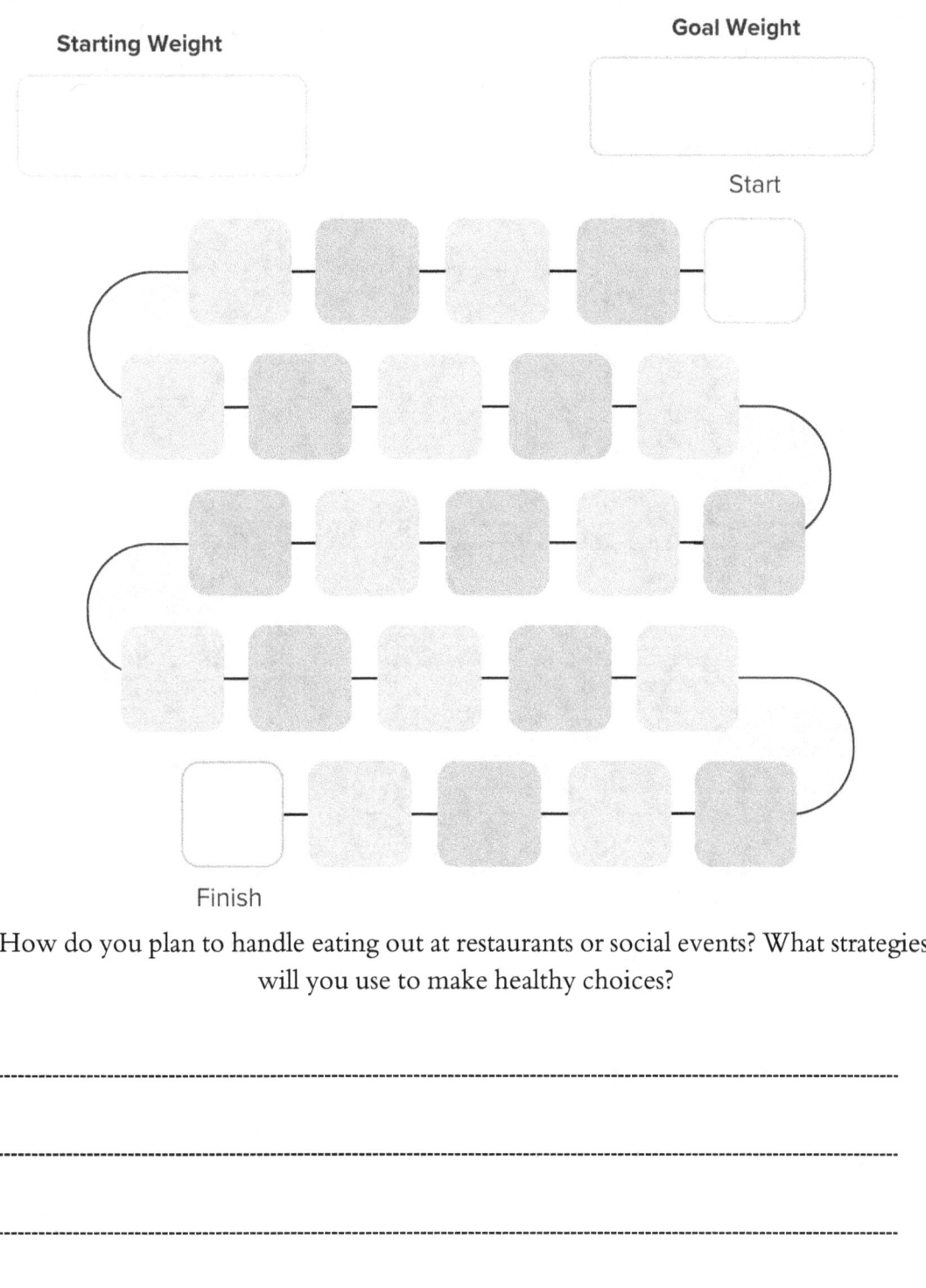

Start

Finish

How do you plan to handle eating out at restaurants or social events? What strategies will you use to make healthy choices?

MONTH.12.

Weight Loss Tracker

Starting Weight

Goal Weight

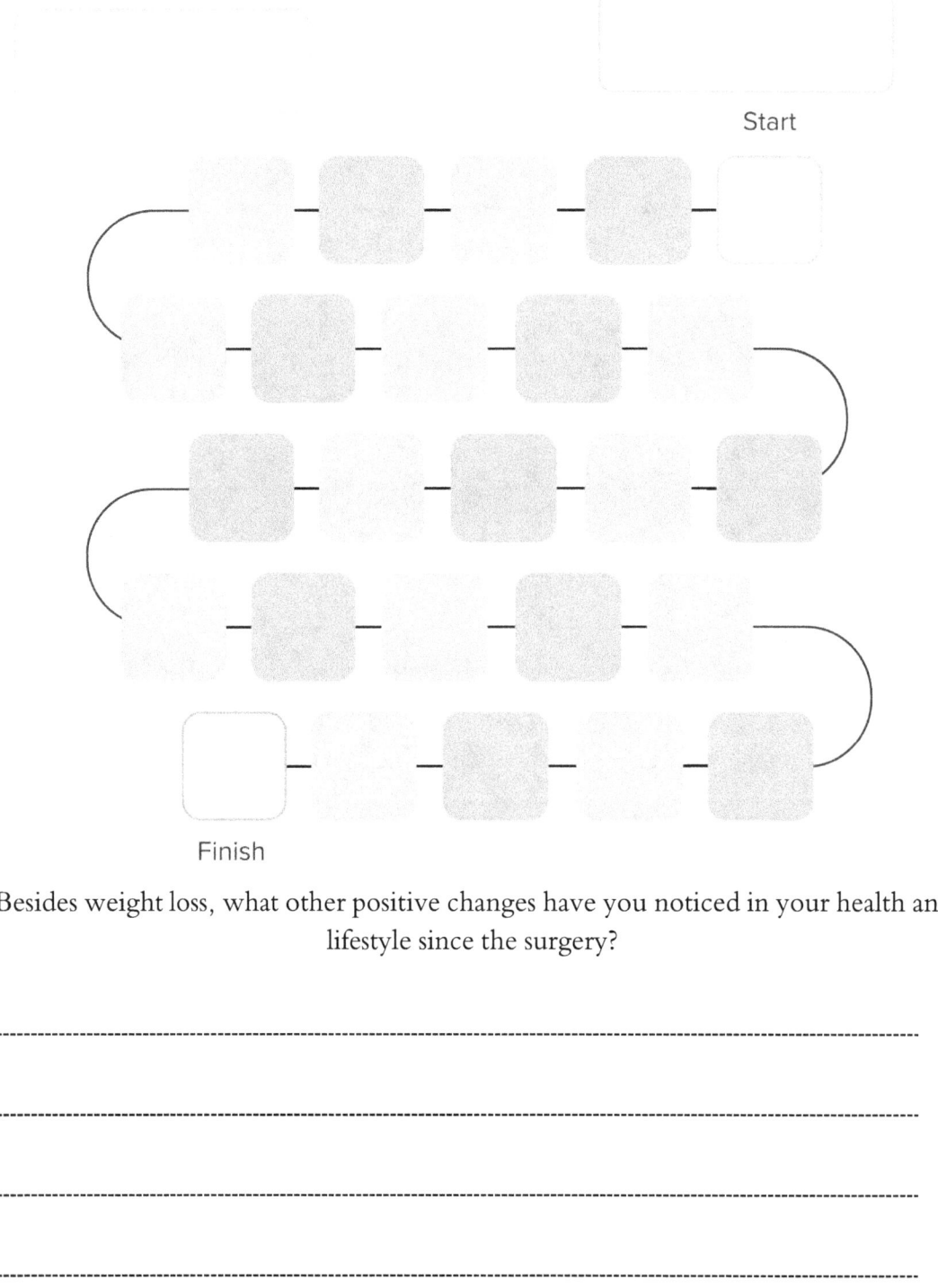

Start

Finish

Besides weight loss, what other positive changes have you noticed in your health and lifestyle since the surgery?

Weight Loss Tracker

Starting Weight

Goal Weight

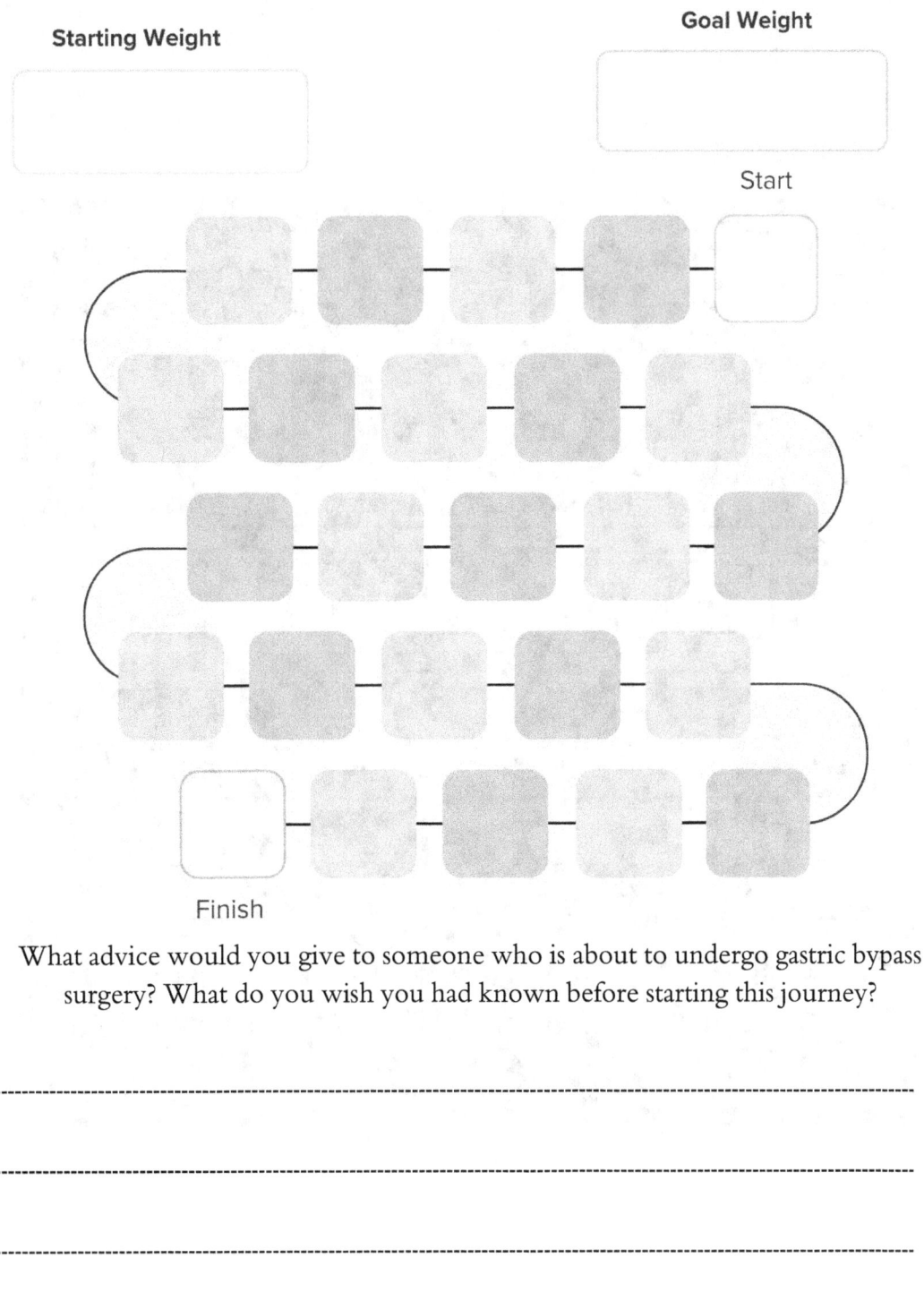

What advice would you give to someone who is about to undergo gastric bypass surgery? What do you wish you had known before starting this journey?

Scan the QR Code to Get Your Special Bonus

www.ingramcontent.com/pod-product-compliance
Lightning Source LLC
Chambersburg PA
CBHW082206220526
45470CB00010B/3066